Analyzing Falls, Pressure Sore and IV Therapy Cases

Patricia Iyer MSN RN LNCC

The Pat Iyer Group
Fort Myers, FL

Analyzing Falls, Pressure Sore and IV Therapy Cases

This product is for sale. Purchase a copy at www.legalnursebusiness.com.

Cover design and layout by Jessica Wilson
Editorial support by Jill Lapinas

Published by
The Pat Iyer Group
11205 Sparkleberry Drive
Fort Myers, FL 33913
908-391-7933
www.legalnursebusiness.com

Legal nurse consultants, collect your valuable
free ebooks at **www.legalnursebusiness.com**.

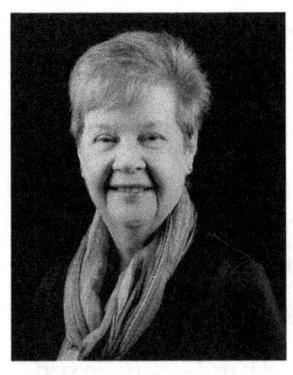

About the Author

PATRICIA W. IYER, MSN RN LNCC

President, The Pat Iyer Group – education for legal nurse consultants at www.legalnursebusiness.com

Fort Myers, FL

Patricia Iyer has been a legal nurse consultant since 1987 when she first began reviewing cases as an expert witness. She achieved national prominence through her texts and many contributions to the legal nurse consulting field. She was the chief editor of *Legal Nurse Consulting Principles and Practices, Second Edition*, the core curriculum for legal nurse consulting. She completed 5 years on the Board of Directors of the American Association of Legal Nurse Consulting including a term as president.

Reach her at patriciaiyer@gmail.com

What Attorneys Say About Pat

Your demeanor and professionalism surely came through to the jury to such an extent that I do not believe defense counsel had any basis to challenge the testimony you were there to offer. The exhibits you prepared were most useful during your trial testimony and we were able to refer to these exhibits at various other times during the trial through other witnesses. When you arrived with eight loose leaf binders indexed and coded, it became clear that the fees we paid for your preparation of this case were well justified by all the time it obviously took to organize and review these materials.
Alan Zibelman Esq. of Philadelphia

I wanted to send you a note to thank you for your efforts in the above matter. I was quite impressed with your high level of preparedness, and also with your very good communication skills with the jury.
Michael Barrett, Esq. of Wilentz, Goldman & Spitzer, Woodbridge, NJ

On behalf of my client and myself, I would like to take this opportunity to thank you for all of your cooperation and professionalism in assisting us with this case that has been successfully resolved. It is due to your efforts and cooperation that provided me the ability to be adequately prepared to take this matter to trial. I would like to thank you for all you have done. I look forward to working with you in the future.
Marc C. Saperstein of Davis, Saperstein and Salomon, Teaneck, NJ

Thanks to you and your staff for all of the help you have given me over the last year in the various medical/legal matters which I am handling. I really appreciate the professional manner in which you deal with my cases and the experts whom you recommend. I have been very pleased with the quality and timeliness of your service. Keep up the good work!
Frances E. Baldo, Jr., Esq. of Yannocone and Baldo, Media, PA

Your liability report and pre-deposition pointers were the keys to my client's case against the hospital nurses, and your medical research greatly enhanced my understanding of the techniques and complications associated with the unusual surgical procedure employed in this particular case. For these reasons alone, your organization should surely rate five stars in any attorney's book.
Patrick X. Amoresano Esq.

I wanted to thank you, once again, with regard to the excellent work that you did in this case in support of our client. Your evaluation of his medical records and presentation of a very compelling report was, we believe, instrumental in our receiving the full policy limit settlement (note typo in original) of $6,000,000. Defense counsel did comment, prior to settlement, that they found your report to be an impressive summary of the medical evidence in the case and description of the pain Mr. * endured following the incident and during the course of his treatment. Once again, we wish to thank you and your staff for your assistance in this matter.
Kenneth Fulginiti, Esq. of Duffy & Associates, PA

The exhibits you provided charting her intramuscular injections, from her admission date through her discharge date, with the medication key chart were extremely helpful. Your reading of the pain medication chart, and transplanting those readings into dates, times and locations of the intramuscular injections, and transposing them into a female anatomy was equally impressive. (The Suffolk County case settled on the fourth day of trial for $625,000.)
Louis Solimano Esq., of New York

Table of Contents

Introduction

This text is a practical guide to understanding three common areas of liability: falls, pressures sores, and intravenous injuries. These injuries have in common that Centers for Medicare and Medicaid Services (CMS) have labeled them as *never events* which should not happen in health care. The loss of reimbursement for care associated with these conditions has intensified the efforts of hospitals to reduce their incidence. It has also resulted in a useful argument for plaintiff attorneys: "The government says this should not have happened."

Falls, pressure sores and intravenous injuries may occur in several areas where nursing care is delivered, and may result in significant consequences, including death.

There are three primary audiences for this material:

- The plaintiff attorney who must understand enough about these injuries to be able to screen cases for merit and know which cases should be further investigated.

- The defense attorney who when faced with a claim involving these kinds of cases, should be able to evaluate the claim to assign the degree of risk and the likelihood of winning the case.

- The legal nurse consultant providing medical guidance in the analysis of the claim, creation of chronologies and timelines, locating expert witnesses and preparing demonstrative evidence.

This text is not a comprehensive discussion of the complexities of the standards of care. It offers an overview of the causes, consequences, treatment, and prevention of falls, pressure sores and intravenous injuries. It provides guidance on how to analyze the liability associated with each type of injury. I hope it will be useful to you.

Acknowledgements

The author appreciates the contributions of these individuals to the material in this book.

Paul N. Bryman, DO, FACOI, AGSF, CMD

Jane Heron, RN, BSN, MBA, LNCC

Diane Krasner, PhD RN CWCN CWS MAPWCA FAAN

Barbara Levin, BSN RN MSCRN ONC LNCC

Sue Masoorli, RN

Deanna Miceli, DNSc APRN FAAN

Falls

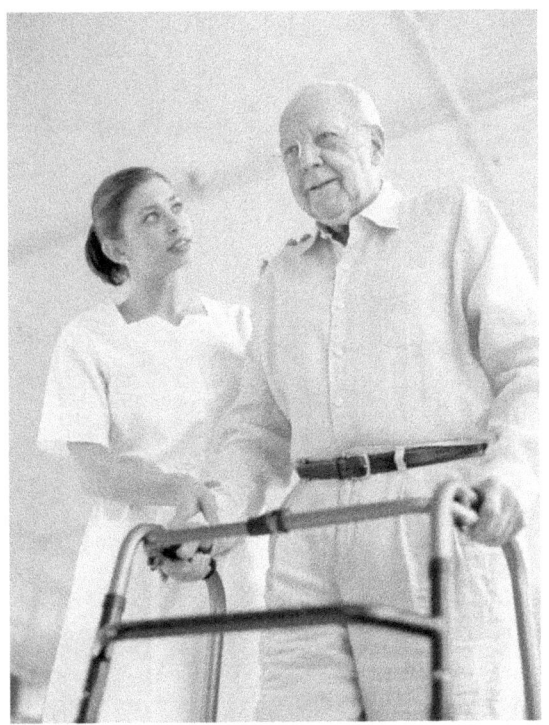

Chapter 1 Why Falls Happen

Definition of a Fall

Inpatient falls and fall-related injuries continue to be the largest category of reported incidents in the acute care setting. They are a frequent cause of lawsuits for both acute and long term care institutions. I have reviewed hundreds of medical records involving falls, either as an expert witness or in the process of supplying experts for falls cases. Falls may also be the basis of personal injury claims related to slippery surfaces. A case may start as a personal injury claim involving a fall, and then evolve into a medical malpractice case related to medical mismanagement of the injuries sustained during a fall.

The technical definition of a fall is any *unplanned* descent to the floor. However, when healthcare providers lower a patient to the floor, they may not consider it a fall. An adult with osteoporosis may suffer a fracture after any impact with a hard surface. Osteoporotic bones are already thinned and fragile. Elderly white females are at highest risk for osteoporosis. While falls can affect patients at any age, the most devastating injuries occur to older people.

Many of the healthcare-related falls that result in injury occur in patients who got up unassisted. I have seen healthcare malpractice cases involving falls off a stretcher, an x-ray table, an operating room table, roof or balcony, out of a chair, bed, commode or window, and in the hallway or bathroom. In short, a patient can fall anywhere on the healthcare premises.

An *assisted* fall occurs when the healthcare staff members are with the patients –helping them to walk. If the patient begins to fall, the staff members might be able to stop the fall or lower the patient to the floor. That is still defined as a fall, but in general, usually doesn't result in any injuries.

Falls occur in many settings. In one week, Med League got four calls looking for expert witnesses for falls cases: a young brain injured woman who fell off a treadmill at home while under the care of an aide, an elderly woman who fell getting off an examining table in a doctor's office, a woman who fell in the hospital just before the nurse reached her side, and a man who fell walking out an adult daycare setting.

Cost of Falls

The Centers for Medicare and Medicaid Services (CMS) calculate there are approximately 20 million falls within communities (within and outside of healthcare facilities) each year. One out of 10 of those falls results in serious injury among older adults. The serious injuries include intracranial bleeding, fracture, dislocation, and crush injury. These injuries added billions to our healthcare costs.

CMS defined some falls as a never event or a "serious and costly error in provision of health services that should never happen." CMS refused to pay for medical care necessitated by a never event. Since CMS took that stand effective October 1, 2008, Medicaid and private payors also stated they did not want to reimburse for care related to falls.

When will CMS reimburse for care after a fall? CMS looks at how the hospital classified the fall. Was the fall due to the original diagnosis or was it due to another factor? Was the patient on a stretcher with the side rails up, alert and oriented and decided on his or her own volition to climb off of that stretcher? That fall would be due to the patient's volition and the medical care for the injuries would be reimbursed.

If a patient was post-operative and had some delirium or confusion and fell, the injuries from that fall would not be covered under the assumption that the fall was preventable. If measures were not taken to prevent that fall and the fall occurred, the hospital would not be paid for care rendered as a result of the fall. Judgments about the preventability of a fall can cost a facility thousands of dollars in lost revenue and even more in settlements or verdicts.

Common Reasons Why Falls Occur

Falls occur because of *intrinsic or extrinsic factors*. Intrinsic are medical or internal factors. Extrinsic are environmental or external factors. Let's look at some reasons within either one of those two categories. A fall may be caused by a combination of the two kinds of factors. For example, a person with poor vision and unsteadiness may fall over a chair left in her way.

Intrinsic Factors
Elimination

Many falls are associated with a patient getting out of bed to go to the bathroom. Intravenous fluids and some medications may increase the frequency of urination. Laxatives, bowel preparations and diarrhea may result in the patient rushing to the bathroom. Some patients fall because they are unable to wait for a staff member to assist them to the bathroom, or their call bell is not responded to quickly enough. I reviewed several cases as an expert witness involving patients who asked for help getting out of bed; no one responded to their light. They got up without help and fell. Some patients fall because they are unable to walk the distance to the bathroom, and do not have a commode at the bedside. They may slip in their own urine or feces.

Visual Impairment
Visual impairment is one of the leading risk factors for falling. It affects people of all ages. Visual problems run the gamut from reliance on glasses to legal blindness (defined as corrected visual acuity in the better eye of 20/200 or worse).

Three percent of persons over the age of eighty-five in the United States are legally blind; approximately 25 percent of nursing home residents are legally blind. Blindness is caused by diabetes, glaucoma, hypertension, cataracts, trauma, and arteriosclerosis, among other factors. An older person needs approximately three times as much light as a twenty-year-old needs. Moving out of a darkened room into bright light causes visual difficulty because the older eye adapts more slowly to changes in illumination. Visual changes such as this increase the risk of injury for elders coming out of a darkened bedroom into a bathroom.

Age-related macular degeneration (AMD) is the number one cause of vision loss and legal blindness in adults over 60 in the U.S. As our population ages, and the baby boomers advance into their 60s and 70s, we will see a virtual epidemic of AMD. Although it rarely causes total blindness, age-related macular degeneration robs those affected of their sharp central vision and can dim contrast sensitivity and color perception. It destroys the clear, "straight ahead" central vision necessary for reading, driving, identifying faces, watching television, doing fine detailed work, safely navigating stairs and performing other daily tasks we take for granted. Peripheral vision may not be affected, and it is possible to see "out of the corner of your eye".

The impact of AMD can be devastating to those who were independent and active prior to the onset of this cruel impairment. Their visual world gradually diminishes into a vague blur, making ordinary daily activities challenging. Cataracts, glaucoma, diabetic retinopathy, stroke, and retinal tears also impact vision. Any of these conditions may be present in the elderly and cause a fall.

Metabolic Changes
A patient may have a change in blood pressure when he stands up; he may not have any symptoms. He may be sitting in a seat, perhaps in the hospital or nursing home. When he stands up, the blood rushes to his feet. He may not have the built in physiological mechanisms to tell him that he is dizzy. He may fall immediately to the ground.

The drop in blood pressure is called *postural hypotension* or *orthostatic hypotension*. It is caused by physiological factors and the side effects of some medications. When the patient changes position, the blood pressure plummets. Detection of the risk of this happening is something healthcare providers have directly under their control. When a patient is frail and comes into the hospital or nursing home, the staff can quickly assess her blood pressure when supine, sitting and standing, and document that. If they detect a significant difference in blood pressure in different positions, and recognize this huge risk factor for falling, they can make some modifications in diet, fluids, and in different adaptive modalities. For example, antiembolic stockings increase the blood flow to the heart. Just by doing some very simple maneuvers the risk for falling can be lowered.

When I worked on the medical surgical nursing units as a staff nurse, I routinely got a patient from a flat to a sitting position. (This is called *dangling* because the feet dangle off the edge of the mattress.) I'd count to ten before helping the patient stand up. (The nurse should count with the patient as a simple reminder of a safety technique.) Then I stood the patient up and stood next to the patient and asked, "How do you feel? Do you feel dizzy? Do you feel okay?" I gave the patient those few moments of adjustment before getting the patient up to a standing position. This simple technique can make all the difference between being upright or being on the floor.

Patients may fall because of a heart arrhythmia. For example, the person may be in the hospital because of a need for a pacemaker. The patient falls because of the irregularity and the impaired conduction of the heart. The patient may fall due to aortic stenosis, coronary artery disease, carotid sinus syndrome and anemia.

The patient may fall as a result of an acute illness, such as a urinary tract infection, pneumonia, sepsis and other factors. She may become deconditioned, losing muscle mass and strength, from being in bed for a long time. A patient may fall because of cervical or lumbar stenosis causing spinal cord compression or spasticity.

The long standing alcoholic may develop cerebellar disease. The diabetic may develop peripheral neuropathy.

Gait and Balance

Another major risk factor for falls has to do with gait and balance. An impairment in this area is a huge medical reason why people fall. Impairments can be caused by weakness, side effects of medications, lingering effects of anesthesia, fever, and deconditioning. Gait disorders are displayed when the patient takes small steps, walks slowly, has a weak leg, or needs to use a walker, cane or wheelchair to move about. Gait can be affected by contractures from a stroke. The patient may have a gait disorder from normal pressure hydrocephalus, Huntingdon's chorea or Parkinson's disease. She may have musculoskeletal reasons for an impaired gait:

- Foot disorders
- Contractures
- Arthritis and joint deformities
- Muscle weakness

Balance may be affected by inner ear lesions, subdural hematomas, and brain tumors. The patient may show increased swaying and have a decreased ability to adjust when his balance is challenged. The physical therapy notes may describe the patient's *static* and *dynamic balance*. Static balance refers to the ability of the patient to stand upright without swaying. Dynamic balance refers to the ability to stand upright and walk without swaying.

If the healthcare providers do a proper assessment, they will detect the impairment. A simple "get up and go" test is performed when the healthcare provider asks a patient to independently stand up and walk. The provider watches the person walk down the hallway or walk and turn and sit. The provider critically analyzes the patient's gait and balance. The physician, physicians assistant or nurse practitioner may order physical therapy if there is an abnormality. The patient may be unable to maintain upright balance, lean to one side or drag a leg. Or the provider can order that the patient be allowed out of bed with assistance or with supervision or to be kept on bed rest.

The nurses must also assess the patient's ability to walk or sit in a chair, and use judgment in providing the appropriate amount of assistance. If the patient is allowed out of bed with help, for example, the nurse is in the best position to determine if the patient needs one or two caregivers' help. There's a common scenario that I have seen in several cases where the allegation is that the patient needed more physical assistance than was provided. The big issue is how many people attempted to walk the patient — how many people were needed versus how many people were actually involved in that ambulation?

Falls in the bathroom raise the question of whether the patient should have been left alone in the bathroom. Was that a safe decision or a reasonable judgment under the circumstances? The analysis of cases often hinges on whether the fall was foreseeable given the circumstances and the evidence of the patient's capabilities. Safety considerations override privacy needs.

Examining rooms in clinics and healthcare providers' offices may be the sites of falls. Elderly or weak individuals may fall because they were not be given the assistance they needed to safely get off the examining table.

Sudden Loss of Consciousness

Patients can suddenly lose consciousness for a variety of reasons. Either as an expert witness or at the request of an attorney looking for an expert, I have worked on several cases involving patients who fainted after blood was withdrawn. In one case, a young girl fell face forward off a stretcher. In a second, a patient injured his back as he slumped off of a chair. A patient may fall during a transient ischemic attack (sudden episode of loss of consciousness) or as a result of being dehydrated or having heat stroke.

A tragic outcome occurred to a young man who donated blood. He stood up after being properly assessed and he denied dizziness or feeling light headed. He started walking out of the facility; he passed out and hit his neck on the way down and became a high quadriplegic. From a plaintiff perspective, there were enormous damages but the staff in this blood center had properly assessed him.

If you ever see the Red Cross staff drawing blood, their patients are always laying down because they know that there's a high risk of fainting. The person who is drawing the blood is responsible for the safety of the patient. It's the person who's drawing the blood who's absolutely responsible to assess the patient before, during, and after for fainting.

Certainly the patient should be in a safe environment, in a seat, in a full chair. If the patient has a fainting history, he or she should be lying down. But some people don't come and say "I'm a fainter", even if the nurse asks them. They're not willing to answer that question. The nurse needs to be sure that the patient is safe from a potential fall. If the patient is sitting on a stool or at the edge of the table and she faints, surely there's an increased risk of her falling off the chair or off the table. But if she is in a protected position and faints, she faints into the chair or the bed. That prevents the injuries that can occur from a fall. Patients may sustain broken arms, shoulders, jaws, and concussions.

A patient may also fall because of a stroke, heart attack, or seizure. A patient may fall because his blood sugar has dropped. If a patient skips a meal or is on a long acting medication for diabetes management and doesn't eat at regular intervals, he or she can succumb very easily to hypoglycemia. Hypoglycemia can cause changes in levels of consciousness where the person can move from a level of alertness to comatose very quickly if he does not receive glucose given either by mouth or intravenously. The hypoglycemic patient may have a seizure.

Epileptics may fall. In many states, epilepsy is a condition that has to be reported to the motor vehicle division because of the risk for seizing and so forth. As a result of the seizure a person can have a change in level of consciousness or fall to the ground, and that's something that typically has no liability. It's so spurious and hard to predict. However, there is a caveat to that. Consider a case involving an epileptic patient who had a seizure and fell. It was known that she had epilepsy and it was known that her drug levels were too low. The physician group and the nurse practitioner group did not do anything to raise the drug level, resulting in a fall. That situation may have liability.

Dementia

Patients who are confused may fall because of an inability to follow instructions or ask for help in getting up. Healthcare providers evaluate whether a patient is confused or *oriented times 3* — does she know her name, the date, and where she is? *Oriented times 4* adds the element of refers to knowing the events leading up to right now. Confusion may be temporary or permanent. Confusion is associated with Alzheimer's disease, head injuries, brain tumors, side effects of medications, and other factors. Alzheimer's disease tends to have a slow onset. It is a chronic and progressive deterioration of white matter of the brain. The white matter of the brain is responsible for high critical thinking, which we use when we pay bills, answer the phone, drive, and perform certain tasks of daily living.

A person with moderately advanced Alzheimer's can still talk and tell you her name and shake your hand. She may be able to greet the healthcare staff and say, "Hi, how are you today?" On the surface it seems like there's not a problem; there's nothing the matter. But on further inquiry when we force that person to do other tasks that require more in depth types of short term memory, she's unable to perform. An example is,

"When you have to go to the bathroom, put on your call light and wait for me to come." (Medical records also refer to this request as a three part command: "Go to the bathroom, put on your light and wait for me.") People who are confused may be able to follow a one or two part command – or not at all. The Mini Mental State Exam is a commonly used 30 point test that helps to assess a person's degree of dementia. Any score from 25-30 indicates a normal cognition.

Healthcare providers may attempt to *reorient* a confused patient in the hopes of avoiding an injury. This means the staff member supplies the correct answers to the questions of name, date and location. But it may not be possible to effect a sustained improvement in confusion.

Patients with Alzheimer's disease often wander. They usually are not specifically seeking to exit the building, although they may accidentally get out. They may fall as a result of the wandering or elopement from the building, whether that is a home, assisted living facility, hospital or nursing home. Patients in severe end stages of Alzheimer's disease often lose their ability to walk.

Delirium
Delirium is a more acute and short term problem with often reversible causes. It can be caused by dehydration, inadequate nutrition, visual impairment, severe illness, depression, sleep deprivation, surgery, restraints, hearing deficits, poorly managed pain, and abnormal blood sugar. The presence of a new diagnosis

of delirium during a hospital admission may increase a patient's risk of falling six fold. [1]

Environmental Factors

These are some of the extrinsic or environmental factors that help to create risks for people. An attorney making an inspection of the site of a healthcare fall may look for these factors.

- Are the hallways highly polished and slippery, creating a glaring or hazardous surface? Carpeting or non-glare finishes are safer. Is there extra lighting in the hallway and stairwell?
- Is the furniture beige, pink or gray, making it difficult for the older eye to see? Bright contrasting colors—red, orange and yellow—are easier to distinguish.
- Do the stairs lack hand railings?
- Are there large picture windows open to the view outside allowing glare to overwhelm the scene?
- Are the doorways of the rooms painted in the same color as the wall, or are they in a contrasting color to make them easier to see?
- Is the switch plate the same color as the wall, or is it a contrasting color?

Curbs and Stairs

Many elderly people who have limited strength in their legs will fall going up a curb, such as one on the healthcare facility's property, because they are unable

---

[1] Brooks, P. "Postoperative delirium in elderly patients", *American Journal of Nursing*, September 2012, 38

to lift their legs. They may trip on the curb. (The curb height is between four and five inches.) They may also fall because curbs or stairs do not have a contrasting color. If the curb or stairs were a homogenous color, such as the same color cement without any clear contrasting color, someone could fall going down a curb.

You don't have to have visual problems to fall on stairs without contrast. I'm reminded of an experience I had in a restaurant in New York. The floor of the restaurant was on two different levels. There was a step down; there was no contrast in the pattern of the floor before you got to the step down. The tiles were black and white on both levels. The young woman I was with stumbled because she was looking straight forward and not down. Think of the hazard this kind of pattern would pose for a patient in a healthcare facility.

Dangerous Surfaces
Floors in healthcare facilities may be slippery because of

- Floor wax
- Cleaning solutions
- Spilled water
- Urine or feces

The sidewalks or parking lots of healthcare facilities may be dangerous because of

- Ice
- Water
- Poor lighting
- Poor repair

Key Points

1. A fall may be assisted or unassisted. Injuries tend to be worse if a patient falls when a healthcare provider is not present.
2. An incident in which a patient is lowered to the floor is still considered a fall and must be reported and investigated.
3. A patient may fall because of internal or external factors or a combination of both.
4. Visual impairment, weakness, confusion, and sudden changes of blood pressure are frequent causes of falls.
5. Hazardous surfaces may contribute to falls.

The next chapter focuses on the injuries that result from falls.

Chapter 2 Injuries From Falls

Falls and fall related injuries are common in the elderly population. It is extremely difficult to prevent all falls within healthcare facilities. Here are some possible scenarios of falls that occur in a healthcare facility.

- The staff members hear the sickening sound of a crash as the patient hits the floor. The sound of the fall may be accompanied by the metallic clanging of an IV pole or a wheelchair as it clatters to the floor.
- The nurse is walking the patient to the bathroom when the patient suddenly passes out and falls to the floor.
- The nursing assistants are helping the patient move from the bed to a chair. They lose their grip on the patient and she strikes the floor.

This chapter explores typical injuries resulting from falls.

Post Fall Assessment

The patient is lying on the floor. What occurs in the next few minutes makes the difference between diagnosed and undiagnosed injuries. Who finds the patient becomes enormously important.

Think about the environment in which falls occur and the levels of staff taking care of patients. In most healthcare settings, registered nurses are on the premises. The mix of staff is different in acute versus long term care. In acute care, registered nurses are available during all shifts. In long term care, they may be available for 8 hours a day. Licensed practical nurses are more plentiful.

In acute care, physicians are available 24 hours a day to diagnose injuries after a fall. The physician may be an attending, resident, intern, house officer, hospitalist, or an emergency department physician. In long term care, the attending physicians visit once every one or two months, and rely on the nursing staff to notify them of falls that require medical investigation. Definitive diagnosis of injuries may take place when the resident is sent to the emergency department.

The immediate assessment after a fall should occur within moments after the staff member discovers the patient on the floor (in an unwitnessed fall) or immediately after a fall that occurred in the presence of a staff member. These are the most important elements of an assessment.

- What is the patient's level of consciousness? The patient's orientation is checked is she or he alert and oriented x 4? Can the patient describe the events that led up to the fall? Is the patient confused, groggy, or unconscious? Is there any evidence he or she had a seizure (trauma to the tongue, incontinence)?

- What is the patient's pulse? Is her heart rate very slow? Has she had a cardiac arrest?

- Is there evidence of external injury? Are there lacerations or bones jutting out? Is either leg shorter than the other with the foot pointing outwards? These are signs of a fractured hip.

- Are there signs of a head injury? Scalp lacerations often profusely bleed. The patient's head needs to be palpated for bulging or crackling sounds consistent with a fracture. Many confused elders may fall and hit their head, and may not remember doing so. Even though they have gaping wounds they may not even recall that they hit their head.

- Can the patient move his or her arms? In some tragic cases, patients have become paralyzed after a fall.

The staff members need to carefully move the patient to the bed, supporting the neck. Ideally they use a backboard to protect the spine, rather than a sheet. The immediate assessment of the patient is typically performed by a nurse. Nurses do more focused comprehensive post-fall assessments than any other provider because they're on the nursing unit at the time of the fall.

Depending on the setting, a physician, nurse practitioner or physician's assistant is the next person who examines the patient. This individual does a physical examination, takes a history of the fall, and orders diagnostic tests. The healthcare provider has to rely not only on what the patient says occurred, but also on witness accounts and behavioral change. The provider examines the patient and does further analysis.

In the meantime, the nursing staff should be taking vital signs and looking for trends. Vital signs need to be done at the discretion of the practitioner. The nurses should be

- assessing the patient's pain level,
- providing pain relievers,
- determining if the patient has a change in level of consciousness, and
- questioning the wisdom of continuing to administer anticoagulants (if the patient was on them) with the likelihood of possible bleeding.

Soft Tissue Injuries

Most patients are not harmed by falls. Some suffer soft tissue injuries, which are described below.

Sprains

A sprain is the stretching or tearing of ligaments and other tissues at a joint. Most commonly it may affect a patient's hand or leg.

Classification of Sprains

Grade I   Mild injury; involves overstretching or microscopic tearing but without hemorrhage or increased instability of the involved joint. Swelling may develop later.

Grade II   Moderate injury; involves partial, overt tearing of the ligament with at least some ligamentous continuity remaining; usually immediate pain and swelling with decreased function.

Grade III   Severe injury; total loss of ligamentous continuity, that is, disruption of one or more ligaments or the musculotendinous unit. Pain is immediate but subsides because none of the pain fibers are being stretched. Swelling may be minimal because hemorrhage extravasates (spreads) outside of the area into soft tissues.

Other Soft Tissue Injuries

An **abrasion** is the most common type of open wound. It is characterized by skin that has been rubbed or scraped away. The wound must be carefully cleaned to remove any foreign material imbedded in the skin that might cause traumatic tattooing.

A **laceration** is a cut, usually from a sharp object the patient may fall upon. The edges of the laceration may be smooth as with knife wounds, or jagged, as in excessive stretching. The laceration may be superficial, involving only the skin, or deep with damage below the skin. Lacerations are common in head injuries.

A **stab or puncture wound** is a type of laceration. Stab wounds produce short and narrow tunnels of damage. If the wound is deeper than 2 to 3 cms, it should be packed open to allow for drainage and complete healing. Puncture wounds are deep and narrow and tend to seal at the surface, hiding pockets of infection. If the wound appears heavily contaminated, the opening should be widened for thorough cleaning, debridement and drainage. The patient may suffer a stab or puncture wound by falling onto a sharp object.

An **avulsion** is an injury in which a portion of the skin, and sometimes other soft tissue, is partially or completely torn away. Most require skin flaps. The patient may suffer an avulsion by getting a hand or foot caught in something during a fall.

A **contusion** is a crush injury. Cold is applied, then heat. More serious crush injuries are harder to evaluate at first due to massive swelling. The patient may sustain a contusion by hitting a hard surface.

A **hematoma** is a collection of blood within the tissues. It may develop at the site of a fracture, such as a fractured hip, when blood vessels are torn.

Head Injuries

Head injuries cause some of the most serious outcomes of falls. A patient is at increased risk for intracranial bleeding if she was on an antiplatelet medication such as a blood thinner like warfarin or Coumadin, heparin or Lovenox, or even aspirin. (Low dose aspirin at 81 mg a day taken for a protected period of time provides an antiplatelet effect.) Other falls of great concern occur in people who are very frail, meaning people who have decreased muscle mass. They're typically very thin; when they fall they may not have the same protective mechanisms to extend their arm out to brace the fall. They also don't have the same cushioning. That can lead to problems particularly if their head hits the floor or surface.

I have seen a number of cases involving head injuries in which the nurses did not perform a diligent evaluation of the patient's level of awareness. They mistook unconsciousness for sleeping, which resulted in a large accumulation of blood within the brain.

Follow Up Monitoring and Diagnostic Testing

The nursing and medical staff should continue to monitor the patient, looking for head injuries, assessing pain level, and monitoring for changes in level of awareness, over the next hours to days.

Here is a quick overview about diagnostic testing (based on Clinical Guidelines for head injury listed in the National Guideline Clearinghouse). The Glasgow Coma Score is a nationally known scale that evaluates the patient's ability to talk, move his arms and legs, and respond to pain. The maximum score is 15. The minimum score is 3.

Glasgow Coma Score

Category	Response	Score
Eye Opening	Spontaneous - eyes open spontaneously without verbal or noxious stimulation	4
	To speech - eyes open with verbal stimuli but not necessarily to command	3
	To pain - eyes open with various forms of noxious stimuli	2
	None - no eye opening with any type of stimulation	1
Verbal Response	Oriented - aware of person, place, time, reason for hospitalization and personal data	5
	Confused - answers not appropriate to question but correct use of language	4
	Inappropriate words - disorganized, random speech, no sustained conversation	3
	Incomprehensible sounds - moans, groans, and mumbles incomprehensibly	2
	None - no verbalization, even to noxious stimuli	1

Category	Response	Score
Best Motor Response	Obeys commands - performs simple tasks on command and able to repeat task on command	6
	Localizes to pain - organized attempt to localize and remove painful stimuli	5
	Withdraws from pain - withdraws extremity from source of painful stimuli	4
	Abnormal flexion - decorticate posturing that occurs spontaneously or in response to noxious stimuli	3
	Extension - decerebrate posturing that occurs spontaneously or in response to noxious stimuli	2
	None - no response to noxious stimuli; flaccid	1

Testing Adults for Head Injury

Skull x-rays should be done only if CT (Computerized Tomography) scanning is unavailable and the person has a mild head injury. An immediate CT scan should be done in an adult with any of the following

- Eye opening only to pain or not conversing (Glasgow Coma Score/GCS 12 out of 15 or less)
- Confusion or drowsiness (GCS 13-14 out of 15) followed by failure to improve within one hour of clinical observation or within two hours of injury
- Fracture of base of skull, depressed skull fracture, and/or suspected penetrating injuries

- A deteriorating level of consciousness or new focal neurological signs
- Full consciousness (GCS 15 out of 15) with no fracture, but with other symptoms (e.g. severe and persistent headache or two distinct episodes of vomiting)
- History of coagulopathy (clotting or bleeding disorder; taking blood thinners) and loss of consciousness, amnesia, or any neurological features

A CT scan may be performed within 8 hours in an adult who is otherwise well, but has any of the following

- Age over 65 (with loss of consciousness)
- Clinical evidence of a skull fracture (e.g. boggy scalp hematoma) but no clinical features indicative of an immediate CT scan
- Seizure activity
- Significant retrograde amnesia (greater than 30 minutes)
- Dangerous mechanism of injury (pedestrian struck by motor vehicle, occupant ejected from motor vehicle, significant fall from height) or significant assault (e.g. blunt trauma with a weapon)

In adults with a GCS less than 15, who have indications for a CT scan, the cervical spine (neck) should also be scanned. This should include the cervical spine to T4 (Thoracic) images.

Testing of Children (Under 16 Years Old)

The provider involved in the diagnosis of a child with a head injury should order immediate CT scanning for

- GCS equal to or less than 13 in the Emergency Department
- Witnessed loss of consciousness of over 5 minutes
- Suspicion of open or depressed skull injury or tense fontanelle (space between bones of infant's skull)
- Focal neurological deficits (such as a seizure or a weak arm or leg)

Any sign of a basal skull fracture may also warrant an immediate CT scan. CT scanning within 8 hours should be considered for the following:

- Presence of any bruise, swelling, or laceration greater than 5 cm on the head
- Post-traumatic seizure, with no history of epilepsy or reflex anoxic seizure (caused by a temporary interruption in the blood supply to the brain which can be caused by sudden unexpected stimulus, such as pain or fear)
- Amnesia lasting greater than 5 minutes
- Clinical suspicion of non-accidental head injury
- A significant fall
- Age less than 1 year with GCS less than 15 in emergency department
- Three or more episodes of vomiting
- Abnormal drowsiness (slowness to respond)

MRI (Magnetic Resonance Imaging) is usually

only done when patients have mental status changes that are unexplained by CT scan findings. An MRI can be more sensitive than CT scans in identifying non-hemorrhagic (no bleeding) diffuse axonal lesions.

Indications for Admission to the Hospital

An adult should be admitted to the hospital if the

- Patient's level of consciousness is impaired (GCS less than 15 out of 15)
- Patient is fully conscious (GCS is 15) but has any indication for an immediate CT scan (if the CT scan is normal and there are no other indications for admission, the person may be considered for discharge)
- Person has significant medical problems
- Person has social problems and can't be supervised by a responsible adult

A person may require neurosurgical assessment, monitoring, or other care management if there is

- Persistent coma (GCS is equal to or less than 8 out of 15) after initial resuscitation
- Persistent confusion for more than four hours
- Deterioration in the level of consciousness after admission (a sustained drop of one point on the motor or verbal GCS scales, or two points on the eye opening scale)
- Focal neurological signs
- Seizure without full recovery
- Compound depressed skull fracture
- Definite or suspected penetrating injury
- A cerebrospinal fluid (CSF) leak or other sign of a basal skull fracture

A delay in diagnosis or a failure to diagnose intracranial bleeding may result in death. The most serious consequence is blood building up in the brain, causing the brain to shift downward (herniation) and press on the brain stem. This interferes with vital functions and results in death.

Fractures
Open and Closed

Fractures are usually described according to their site, the extent of the fracture, the configuration, the relationship of the fragments and the complications. Fractures are classified as *open* or *closed*. An open fracture is also known as a compound fracture, where the bone actually penetrates through the soft tissue to the skin. It may be accompanied by a crush injury, which results in the tissues literally being smashed. A closed fracture is also known as a simple fracture which means that there is no contact between the bone and the skin.

Open fractures are the ones that place the patient at a higher risk for developing an infection. Those are the fractures that will require the patient be stabilized and brought to the operating room, sooner instead of later. The orthopaedic surgeon will need to do an irrigation and debridement to reduce the contaminants in the wound. The surgeon also needs to evaluate the injury and determine how and when to close the wound.

An x-ray of a *spiral* fracture would show a break that goes around the bone in a spiral fashion. This is a twisting injury and might happen if a patient caught her foot in something and twisted her leg as she fell. There are also segmental fractures, which occur when two or more separate fractures of the same bone result in the formation of a central fragment. There could be a fracture at the top of the bone and at the bottom of the bone, for example.

Impacted fractures occur when broken bone edges are wedged together.

Comminuted fractures occur when great force is applied to the bone, as the bone is literally shattered into many pieces. Think of the bone like a piece of hard candy that shatters into many pieces. It produces three or more fragments.

Linear fractures are parallel to the long axis on the bone, whereas *transverse* fractures occur when the bone is snapped across.

A *compression* fracture results when one bone is forced against another, such as when a patient's vertebrae are crushed. This may happen with falls or direct blows.

A *burst* fracture occurs in the spine when pieces of vertebrae are forced backwards into the spinal canal and may result in paralysis.

While all fractures are painful, some are more painful than others. Fractured ribs and pelvic fractures tend to be very painful because these areas cannot be effectively immobilized.

Fractures associated with tissue trauma are more painful. Hand fractures are more painful due to the multiple nerve endings in the hands, as well as the associated swelling.

Classification of Open Fractures

Type I Wound < 1 cm
        Moderately clean, minimal contamination
        Fractures—simple transverse or oblique with
        skin pierced by bone spike
        Minimal soft tissue damage

Type II Wound > 1 cm
        Moderate contamination
        Fractures—moderate comminution/crush
        injuries
        Moderate soft tissue damage (flaps or
        avulsion)

Type   High degree of contamination
III   Fractures—severe comminution and
        instability
        Extensive soft tissue damage involving
        muscle, skin, and neurovascular structures
        Traumatic amputations

IIIA   Soft tissue coverage of fracture is adequate
        Fractures—segmental or severely comminuted

IIIB   Extensive injury to or loss of soft tissue,
        periosteal stripping, and exposure of bone
        Massive contamination
        Fractures—severe comminution

IIIC   Any open fracture associated with arterial
        injury that must be repaired regardless of
        degree of soft tissue injury

Complications of fractures include nonunion, malunion, traumatic arthritis, heterotopic ossification (excessive bony growth), and osteomyelitis (bone infection). All can be associated with chronic pain and are difficult to treat.

The types of fractures that result from a fall depend on how the patient fell. Did she fall forward? In that case, the healthcare providers need to consider any type of wrist fractures and also assess if there is a frontal head injury. A patient who knows she is about to fall may put out her arms to brace herself and stop her body from hitting the floor. This could result in a wrist fracture, also called a Colles fracture. This is a break of the end of the radial bone or the scaphoid bone.

I watched a woman literally fracture her shoulder and wrist when she fell at my feet at an airport. She was talking and not paying attention to where she was going and tripped over my suitcase. She slammed her shoulder into the bag checker's podium and braced herself with her wrist. Her wrist bent at an unnatural angle and flopped down. This is a typical Colles fracture. The limited blood supply in the wrist affects healing. Casting is usually the treatment of choice because the physician wants to limit the shearing forces that would prevent the healing. This type of fracture may result in a non-union of the bones.

If a patient falls backwards, oftentimes hip fractures or posterior head injuries occur. Falls from a height, such as off a bed, may result in hip, elbow and skull fractures.

More than 300,000 elderly adults experience a hip fracture each year. Femoral neck fractures are a very common type of hip fracture. They are seen more often in women and the frail elderly. *Intertrochanteric* fractures occur when the fracture is between the trochanters or the knobby areas at the top of the femur. *Sub-trochanteric* means "below" or below the lesser trochanter. Intertrochanteric and the sub-trochanteric fractures are more commonly seen in males and the more active elderly because it takes a greater trauma or force to cause those injuries.

Facial Fractures

Patients who fall face forward are at risk for facial fractures. The type of fracture is labeled based on the part of the face that is injured.

- LeFort I transverse or horizontal fracture that involves the front teeth up to the nose
- LeFort II pyramid shaped fracture that encompasses the central portion of the maxilla (cheek) up to the nose
- LeFort III separation of facial bones from the cranium (skull)

Facial fractures may result in deformity and scarring. A significant amount of surgical reconstruction with plates may be needed to restore appearance.

Muscle Strength

Limb or spinal fractures may result in loss of strength. Weakness is graded using the scale below. Several different scales for grading muscle strength exist. A common numerical scale follows:

- Grade 5 or normal

- can hold or move body part against gravity with maximum resistance
- Grade 4 (good)
  - can hold or move body part against gravity with minimum to moderate resistance
- Grade 3 (fair)
  - can hold or move body part against gravity only
- Grade 2 (poor)
  - can move body part through range of motion against gravity with support/assistance
- Grade 1 (trace)
  - cannot move body part at all, but some muscle contraction can be felt
- Grade 0 (zero)
  - no evidence of muscle contraction

Surgical Repair

At times, patients are too unstable medically to take them directly to the operating room for surgery for fractures. Some patients will need medical and/or cardiac clearance prior to going to the operating room. In general, orthopaedic surgeons prefer to take patients to the operating room as soon as the patient is stable. The longer the patient waits, the more pain and suffering occurs.

An open reduction of a fracture is accomplished by using nails, pins, plates, screws, or wires to hold the fracture pieces together. You will hear the term, ORIF which is an Open Reduction Internal Fixation. That's the type of procedure that will be used to repair fractured hips or limbs. The surgeon may use a nail, a pin, or a hip compression screw. Or maybe the individual will need a total hip replacement, which means replacing the femoral head and the acetabulum cup, for example.

Conservative Treatment

Some nonambulatory patients do not require surgery for a fracture. Perhaps the fracture was non-displaced; perhaps the patient is stable or not able to walk. My neighbor is a paraplegic who fell out of bed and fractured the tibial plateau of his knee. He received a leg brace instead of surgery. Sometimes conservative treatment is the chosen route for those patients who have dementia. Although pain and suffering are consequences of conservative treatment, the risk of bringing patients to surgery may outweigh the benefits.

Conservative treatment may consist of Bucks traction for a fractured leg. Bucks traction is accomplished by putting the foot into a boot that is attached to weights. It helps to decrease the muscle spasms while immobilizing the leg. Bucks traction also reduces pain and may be used for individuals who are waiting to go to the operating room.

A closed reduction of a fracture involves manipulating the leg to place the bones back into alignment. A closed reduction is actually a manipulative reduction at the fracture site without using an incision. For example, a fractured hip is made up of a femoral head and acetabulum. The hip joint is a ball and a socket joint; think of a baseball and a glove. The baseball is out of its glove. The physicians will utilize force, often medicating the patient to help relax them, to help pull that extremity and put it back into its socket.

A plaintiff who fractured her leg testified about the orthopaedist's attempt to do a closed reduction in the ER. Her statement was, "All the babies that I had and all of the labor that I have undergone in my lifetime was nothing like having a closed fracture being reduced." She received no anesthesia or pain reduction medication beforehand. It is unusual for a patient to undergo this type of painful procedure without anesthesia.

Factors Influencing Post Injury Recovery

Older people tend to have poor outcomes after a fall has occurred. They often have other health issues. They may have osteoporosis (softened bones); they may have osteopenia, which is a de-mineralization of the bone. Eight million women and two million men suffer from osteoporosis. Fifty percent of all women and twenty five percent of all men will have a fracture after the age of 50.

A hip fracture is an acute event that can have major lifestyle changes. Only about 50 percent of the elderly who have sustained a hip fracture will return to their pre-fracture level of function. In addition, 25 percent of elderly patients who fracture their hips die within three months. Thirty-five percent will die within a year. Death is usually related to a variety of complications that can occur as a result of a hip fracture. The typical downward spiral after a fracture often results in immobility, which is associated with pneumonia, pressure sores and death. Those who do not die may suffer from permanent disability, inability to carry out independent activities, or inability to walk independently.

The elderly are at particular risk for complications after a fall because of the risk factors already mentioned: osteoarthritis, decrease in vision, orthostatic hypotension, gait alterations and instability with mobilization. Some patients do not have the physiological capability of regaining mobility.

Postoperative Complications

Operative treatment carries risks. Aside for the usual risks of anesthesia, bleeding and nerve damage during surgery, the *postoperative* period also carries risks.

Delirium

In the previous chapter, I mentioned delirium as a cause of falls. In the postoperative phase patients may develop delirium. This is an abrupt onset or transient changes and disturbances in cognition. The patient who had general anesthesia may be a little confused after surgery and may need reminders and reorientation in the initial postoperative phase. These individuals may become confused; they forget that they had a fracture. They may be unaware of their surroundings, climb out of bed and fall onto the floor and end up with a second fractured hip or a head injury. Even worse, some of the patients who are on anticoagulation, may fall, hit their head and suffer an intracranial bleed.

Some facilities utilize psychiatric nurse clinicians to identify those patients who are having post-operative delirium. The clinicians advise how to treat those individuals.

Blood Clots

There is a risk of accumulation of blood clots in the legs of patients after surgery. Several factors contribute to the development of clots, including immobility, a genetic predisposition for clotting, and blood vessel wall damage that could be due to a trauma or surgery. Clots that develop in the arm are sometimes associated with intravenous catheters. The risk factors either singly or collectively can contribute to the development of deep vein thrombosis. The goal is to prevent the thrombosis, a clot, from breaking off and traveling up to the lung to cause a host of other problems including a respiratory arrest and/or death. Thus many orthopaedic surgeons utilize a variety of modalities for anti-coagulation after surgery. There are some surgeries in which anticoagulation may not be used in the postoperative period.

Getting patients out of bed and walking soon after surgery helps to prevent deep vein thrombosis. Many physicians order antiembolism stockings and pneumoboots (that inflate and deflate to stimulate circulation). Paradoxically, the pneumatic boots, which are connected to a device that inflates and deflates the boots, have been found to be associated with a higher risk of falls in people. This is a particular problem at night time because of the risk of postoperative delirium or confusion coupled with an attempt to get out of bed without help.

Patients commonly go home after orthopaedic surgery with some type of anti-coagulation medication for 14 days to 21 days. This depends on their diagnosis.

Pneumonia
Patients who have undergone anesthesia and are on bed rest are at risk for pneumonia. Patients in the critical care unit who are dependent on ventilators after orthopaedic surgery are at risk high risk for ventilator

associated pneumonia (VAP). This is such a well-recognized risk now that there is a series of protocols to reduce the risk of this complication. These include prevention of peptic ulcer disease, elevation of the head of the bed, and a sedation vacation (periodically stopping sedation).

Nursing care of non-ventilated patients, who make up the majority of patients after hip surgery, includes

- Asking alert and cooperative patients to use incentive spirometry to inhale and exhale to expand their lungs.
- Having the patient do some coughing and deep breathing every hour while awake.
- Monitoring the patient's oxygen saturation level with a clip placed on the finger. (Normal is 95-100%.)
- Listening to the patient's lungs for the quality of the patient's breath sounds. Are there diminished breath sounds? Are the lungs clear? Does the patient have rales or crackles? The presence of rales would indicate that there is fluid in the lungs. Patients with a smoking history have a higher risk of post-operative pneumonia.
- Assessing the patient's vital signs because pneumonia is often associated with an elevated temperature. The patient may have chills or fatigue.

If there is a suspicion of pneumonia, physicians will order a chest x-ray to find out if there is some type of infiltrate. The physician may also order blood and sputum cultures and blood work to look for elevated white blood cells, indicating a possible infection, requiring treatment with antibiotics.

Surgical Site Infections

Surgical site infections used to be commonly accepted as risks of surgery, but there is now increasing emphasis on the preventable nature of these infections. CMS has identified these as never events. Surgical site infections are those areas that become infected in less than 30 days' time from the time of surgery. With regard to a total joint replacement, that definition is a little different, which is that a joint becomes infected within one year of placement.

Was the patient given an intravenous antibiotic in the operating room or pre-operatively? Was that antibiotic administered prior to inflation of a tourniquet?

For example, a patient who fell had an open fracture of the wrist and went to surgery at 11 AM. The tourniquet compressed the arm at 11:10 AM and the surgeon made the incision. Suppose the antibiotic started at 11:20 AM. The antibiotic will not be delivered to that open fracture on that arm because of the tourniquet being on. There needs to be blood flow to bring the antibiotic to the area. So that would certainly be a contributing factor for that infection, in addition to the patient having an open fracture.

In general, patients are given antibiotics pre-op or intra-op prior to the tourniquet placement. They are given a few doses. Some surgeons believe two or three doses should be administered. Other surgeons order antibiotics to be administered for 24 or 48 hours.

A very cold operating room could contribute to surgical site infections. That will decrease the circulation as well. Many surgeons are decreasing the air currents of the operating room by minimizing the amount of people in the operating room suite. This has been an area studied by various researchers.

Hand washing is literally the key to helping protect patients from developing infections. Much attention has been directed to getting healthcare providers to wash their hands before and after touching a patient, with varying degrees of success. Patients who have suffered open fractures and have incisions should not be in a room with somebody that has a gross infection of some sort.

Postoperative monitoring of the patient's oxygen level is important since a low oxygen level can contribute to infections. The surgical site infection rate for orthopedic procedures is very low at only 2 to 3 percent and the rate of infection after a total hip replacement is approximately one percent over the lifetime of a prosthesis.

The incidence of infections is affected by the surgical site and the extent of injury, as well as the patient's ability to fight the infection. Open fractures have a higher incidence of developing an infection. A patient may have very frail health. Perhaps the patient has had a history of infections and pneumonias or perhaps he is a diabetic. That can increase his risk factors as well.

Urinary Tract Infections

It used to be a very common practice to insert a Foley in any patient who was incontinent or at risk for incontinence or might have pain that would prevent easy access to a bed pan or a commode. Patients who have fractured hips experience discomfort getting off and on the bedpan. It is undesirable for a patient to be incontinent of urine and have the urine get onto the surgical site. The healthcare care team now recognizes appropriate and inappropriate uses of Foley catheters.

Appropriate uses of catheters

- Urinary retention
- Need to closely monitor urinary output in a critically ill patient
- Obstruction to the urinary tract below the bladder
- A need to measure urine output accurately in an uncooperative patient (head injury, intoxicated)
- Providing a rapid rate of intravenous fluids to patients with acute renal insufficiency
- Preoperative catheter insertion for patients going directly to the operating room
- Comfort care in the terminally ill patient
- Urinary incontinence posing a risk to the patient from major skin breakdown or protection of a nearby operative site

Inappropriate uses of catheters

- Urinary incontinence without significant skin breakdown
- Convenience for the nursing staff
- Too busy or forgot to remove urinary catheter

The risks of developing a urinary tract infection are directly related to the length of time the catheter stays in. A single catheterization carries a 1-3% risk. A catheter that stays in for fewer than 7 days has a 10-40% risk of promoting infection. A patient who has an indwelling catheter for 28 days or more has a 100% risk of developing an infection. Urinary tract infections, especially with the elderly, can actually be manifested as confusion. In some cases, confusion is the first sign the person has an infection.

Keeping the risks in mind, the standard of care has become removal of the Foley catheter as soon as possible after surgery. Catheters may be in for just 24 hours. The Foley will usually be out by post-op day number two, sometimes post-op day number one in the afternoon. Foleys remain in patients for a much shorter period of time than they have been in the past, which helps to decrease the amount of urinary tract infections that the patients develop in the hospital.

Limitations on Mobility
I've seen a number of cases in which patients who were frail to begin with were not able to regain their mobility after a fracture. Patients who have had total knee or hip replacements may fall in the postoperative period, requiring a redo of their surgery and increased risk of complications. Some frail patients are fearful of falling a second time, and thus walk very rigidly or cautiously while they are undergoing their rehabilitation. Sometimes those are the ones that actually will reinjure themselves because they are so frightened.

Falls with fractures or head injuries can be life altering events. Not only do they affect the patient, they affect the families as well. Perhaps these patients can never live on their own again. They may need to go live with a family member; they may need nursing home placement. Maybe they are 80-years-old; they have been living independently doing very well on their own. Now they have fallen and been injured and are not able to care for themselves. There are a lot of psychosocial issues involved aside from the physical issues and also the family issues.

Death

A patient who falls has an increased risk of dying, particularly if he or she is elderly. Death may be directly related to the fall, such as a catastrophic head injury that results in bleeding, brain shifting and death. A patient may die from a fall from a height. Damage to the cervical spine may result in paralysis of the diaphragm.

Perhaps the patient becomes confused after surgery. Perhaps she tries to climb out of bed and she falls and sustains another injury. Perhaps postoperatively, due to a variety of reasons, she developed pneumonia. The pneumonia may progress. Perhaps she developed bed sores or clots or infections at the surgical site. A patient can experience a cascading of complications. An elderly patient who has these complications, such as pneumonia, may not want to eat that much. This leads to a nutritional deficit, which complicates recovery. She is not able to heal because she is not taking in the proper nutrition. The patient develops an electrolyte issue; maybe she has kidney damage because she is not taking in enough fluids as well. There are so many different things that can occur to these patients.

Key Points

1.   Most falls do not result in injury.
2.   Early detection of injuries from falls is critical for effectively treating the patient.
3.   There are well-defined protocols for the diagnosis of patients who have fallen.
4.   Injurious falls are associated with an increased risk of death, both in the acute phase and during the recovery phase.

The next chapter focuses on prevention. Much misery could be avoided by preventing falls. Prevention is far more complex than you might realize.

Chapter 3 Fall Prevention

Fall prevention is an area that is essential as our population ages and falls continue to be a problem. Governmental, accreditation and professional organizations focus on fall prevention by defining strategies to reduce the incidence of falls. This chapter incorporates some of those efforts.

Risk Factor Assessment

The major key to preventing falls is to try to predict who is going to fall. Once this person is identified, the healthcare team is in a position to carry out measures to reduce the risk of falls. Many healthcare sites use a fall risk assessment. The assessment is usually reviewed on a daily or per patient encounter basis (such as in a clinic or doctor's office) and sometimes every shift in an inpatient facility. The assessment may be informal and based on observation and questioning, or be rooted in a form that is filled out. There is no one universally used risk assessment tool. The facility may use its own form, or one of the more well-known ones, such as the Morse Scale or the Johns Hopkins tool.

The purpose of the assessment is to identify risk factors and to develop an individualized plan of care to prevent a fall. The single most important risk factor is a history of previous falls. The assessment is a nursing tool that examines factors such as

- the mental status of the patient
- the mobility status such as gait/transferring abilities
- the secondary diagnoses

- weakness
- the types of medications the patient is on
- elimination issues (diarrhea, urinary frequency)
- if the patient has an intravenous catheter

Many tools assign points to the risk factors to identify whether the individual is at low, moderate, or high risk for a fall. Some tools do not give a point value.

Once a patient is identified as being at risk for falls, the nursing staff should prepare a care plan that provides individualized interventions to reduce the risk of falls. Many facilities use some form of notification of the staff that the patient is at risk.

- This notification may take the form of a colored arm band. This method notifies everyone who comes in contact with the patient, not just the nursing staff.
- The Ruby Slipper program consists of giving patients red slipper socks to use when they are out of bed to identify that they are at risk for falls.
- The staff may identify a patient at risk for falls by placing a shape, such as star on the hospital door or a green triangle on their door. It is a tool that is utilized so that all staff knows which patients are at risk for a fall.
- In general, patients at risk for falls will be placed closer to the nursing station as well.

The last time I went to visit my mother in a hospital, as I walked down her medical surgical unit I saw that every door had a leaf on it. I assumed this was to identify the falling leaf program or a way of identifying the patient in the room was at risk for falls. However, if the nursing unit is filled with patients at risk for falls, there are not enough beds close to the nursing station. And for this concept to be effective, there has to be someone at the nursing station within hearing distance or able to see the patient trying to get out of bed, and able to intervene in time.

Prevention Techniques

Hourly rounds are used to reduce the risk of falls. Nurses and nursing assistants visit with the patients to assess their needs. The registered nurses are the ones who document on an hourly basis. Nursing assistants may help with whatever the patient's needs are but it is the registered nurse who is doing the documentation on the form or electronic medical record. Facilities' expectations for rounds may vary. Reviewing its policies on hourly rounds and documentation will assist in defining the facility's standards for staff.

Rounds typically address the four "Ps"

- Potty
- Positioning
- Pain
- Possessions - phones, water, glasses, call lights and bedpans within reach.

Falls are reduced when the nursing staff assess patients every hour and identify their needs. The staff assess if the patient needs to utilize the bathroom, commode or a bedpan. Nursing personnel determine if the patient needs assistance with repositioning. The patient's pain level is checked and addressed. The goal is to see if the patient needs pain medication or other types of medication. The staff should make sure the telephone and water pitcher are close.

In some facilities, the staff does rounds every hour in the day time and every two hours in the night time. Hourly rounds result in a significant reduction in call light use, fewer patient falls, and greater patient satisfaction.

Some facilities perform video surveillance of public areas. Typically there will be cameras at entrances and exits of the facility. Privacy considerations discourage use of cameras in patient rooms or bathrooms.

Restraints
Wrist and chest restraints used to be commonly used to tie people to beds or chairs. In the early 1990s, healthcare providers and medical malpractice attorneys alike recognized that restraints carried risks. These include

- nerve damage from patients tugging on wrist restraints
- breathing difficulties from tight chest restraints
- strangulation from chest restraints
- immobility
- deconditioning
- agitation
- acceleration of psychological and functional decline
- other negative effects

Restraints are now used only sparingly, such as to prevent intubated patients from attempting to remove their medical equipment. Alternative measures must be tried first, and the order for a restraint renewed every 24 hours. Patients in restraints are to be carefully monitored, and the restraints periodically removed to put a limb through range of motion.

Alarms and Side Rails

Bed alarms and side rails have been used as measures to prevent falls. Both are controversial. Bed alarms are devices to alert staff that the person is either taking the alarm off or is getting up and changing position without any assistance. The alarm may be placed under the mattress, built into the mattress or consist of a clip placed on the patient's gown. Bed alarms are not a panacea; they're a surveillance device. They are only as good as the ability of the

- staff to get to the room to stop the patient from climbing out of bed,
- staff to hear the alarm, and
- patient to keep the alarm on without removing it.

If the patient was really fortunate there would be a staff member outside the room who would hear the bed alarm and could run in and stop the dangerous behavior before the person got out of bed. Having somebody that close at hand is not always the case.

Some facilities also have chair alarms. The alarm goes off if the individual tries to rise from a chair. The chair alarm has batteries that need to be checked and changed.

I have also seen a fair number of facilities, particularly in long term care, put alarms on the exit doors off of the unit or on the elevator. They may put alarm guards on the patients who are up and walking around. There continues to be a very real concern about elderly people wandering into stairwells of clinical units and then falling downstairs or getting out of the building, with disastrous results.

Side rails, either full length or half the length of the bed, have been relied on to keep patients in bed. Healthcare personnel are now recognizing that these rails are a form of restraint. The Joint Commission, which accredits a large number of facilities in the United States and abroad, views side rails as restraints which require justification and use of alternative measures before they are used. Side rails increase the height of a fall and injury if a patient climbs over them. Patients also can wedge their heads under the rails and strangulate themselves.

Side rails are often discouraged in long term care, except as something the patient can grab to reposition himself. Placing a bed up against a wall to prevent exiting from one side is considered a restraint. A band around the waist or a table in front of the patient is also a restraint. All of these types of devices require careful consideration and their use regulated.

One on one sitters are people who are stationed in the patient's room to watch the patient on a continuous basis. Typically a healthcare facility uses nursing assistants in this role. Some facilities hire sitters who may be from a pool of individuals that will come and literally sit and watch the patient. This type of surveillance is costly to the facility but effective when done properly to protect the patient from impulsively getting out of bed. Some group their confused people, perhaps two in a room, so that one sitter can watch both of them.

Non-nursing assistant sitters do not have any responsibility to touch a patient. So if the patient is trying to climb out of bed, the sitter will summon a nurse to come in. Nursing assistants may touch patients and help them to swing their legs back into the bed if they were sitting on the bedside. All of these things help to keep the patient safe. The sitter will need to be relieved for breaks and is responsible for getting someone to watch the patient during that time.

Facilities may encourage family members to stay with the patient to assume this responsibility. Research findings note that having the family members stay with the patient who is confused helps by adding a degree of familiarity for the patient. The patient is in an unfamiliar environment. Having a familiar person there will help decrease the amount of confusion. In addition, the family helps to keep the patient in the bed. However, this is not a realistic solution for families who live far away or are all working and can't manage to have somebody stay awake all night to sit with Dad to keep him from trying to get out of bed.

Safe Patient Handling

A fall may result in injury to both the patient and the healthcare provider who may be assisting the patient at the time. Safe lifting, moving and transferring patients attack the causes of falls. Many falls result from a healthcare provider not being able to supply the degree of assistance the patient needed. Frail patients who are unsteady on their feet, obese patients, or weak people whose legs give way, are at risk for overwhelming the capabilities of the helper. A careful assessment of the patient's capabilities and risk factors for falls may prevent many falls, but others may result from an unexpected change in the patient's strength.

Many healthcare facilities have invested in equipment to safely move patients. These may include hydraulic lifts, slings that are anchored to the ceiling, chair lifts and other devices. In late 2012, a consensus panel of experts, through the American Nurses Association, released a draft of National Safe Patient Handling Standards for public comment. Once finalized the standards are intended to be used to create policy, laws and regulations to protect healthcare providers and patients from injury. They will encourage best practices in patient handling and mobility and will form part of the foundation of the standards of care for fall prevention.

Environmental Factors

In Chapter 1, I discussed environmental factors and their contribution to falls. Many of these risk factors are well known – poor lighting, slippery floors, or lack of contrast. But other environmental factors are in integral part of the healthcare environment. For example, I worked on a case of a pregnant woman who tripped over a wheelchair that was not properly stored out of the way of traffic. Someone did not take the few seconds needed to fold up the wheelchair. There may be other pieces of equipment that block the patient's path.

Even something as simple as the IV tubing can trip a patient. Long tubing can drag on the floor.

Healthcare facilities must conform to particular and rigorous standards as to how they set up their rooms. Grab bars, emergency cords, the height of toilet seats, night lights and other elements are regulated.

Medical malpractice attorneys who litigate cases recognize that these are very common events in the elderly populations and that you can't keep people in bed 100 percent of the time. In fact it's not desirable to keep people immobilized because of the other complications that can occur. As long as you have got a population that's up and walking around there is a risk of falls occurring. This leads to the need, therefore, to try to keep the environment as safe as possible for the people who are elderly, confused or demented, who are wandering around settings such as hospitals and long term care units.

Individualized Factors

Risk factors for falls are individualized and thus dictate the preventative measures. Some people fall because they impulsively get out of bed to go to the bathroom without asking for help. Some people fall because they wear slippery socks. Some fall because they get dizzy when they stand up too quickly. Some fall because they are weak. Did the fall occur because of dementia, a visual impairment or gait impairment? There are nuances that are very unique to each person as to why he is falling. The focus shifts from how the fall occurred to why it occurred. Did the nurses identify the specifics through an individualized assessment and then target a specific plan? Until nurses assess the individual's risk factors, they cannot effectively prevent falls.

A root cause analysis gets at the "why" a fall occurred. It looks at all the factors and the variables and it helps to hone in on the most likely factors associated with the fall. Once a patient has fallen, the healthcare team should evaluate the factors that lead to the fall so they can modify the plan of care to prevent future falls.

The next chapter addresses this as part of the standard of care.

Key Points

1. Risk factor assessment is designed to systematically consider the factors most commonly associated with falls.
2. Facilities use different methods to communicate a patient's risk for falls.
3. Restraints are used as a last resort, and then for time limited periods.
4. Sitters and alarms are among the strategies used to reduce the incidence of falls.

The next chapter provides guidance on developing a falls case.

Chapter 4 Liability for Falls

I'd like you to envision you are sitting in a plaintiff's law firm. You may be an attorney or legal nurse consultant responsible for answering calls. The phone rings and the voice at the other end of the lines says, "My mother was in the hospital and fell out of bed and broke her hip." What are some of the questions that you should be asking the caller?

Aside from the questions that help you determine the statute of limitations, the questions that elicit clinical details should help you gather as much information as possible about the circumstances of the fall.

- Why was the patient in the hospital?
- How old was she?
- What was her physical and mental condition before the fall?
- Was she independent or did she need assistance?
- What kinds of assistance did she need?
- Did the nursing staff tell the daughter her mother was at risk for falling?

If the caller is a very astute kind of well-educated consumer, you might hear, "Yes, my mom was assessed for a risk and she had *no* risk factors to fall. They told me she has no risks and I have a piece of paper here that says, "She has no risk for falls".

Important Details

Some of the questions that follow can be answered based on the family member's knowledge. Others require review of the medical records.

1. What was the mental status of the patient? What was happening to her? Was she confused? Was this a change? There are many reasons why an older person can develop confusion. It can be caused by a transfer to a new environment or new medications that act through the central nervous system. Knowing the person's mental status can provide some important clues as to what might have transpired.

2. What were the physician's orders? Were the orders written for the patient to be on bed rest only, unable to get out of bed or out of bed with assistance? Ask the caller about the patient's prior level of mobility and independence.

3. Had the patient ever fallen before? Statistically, people who have fallen once are more likely to fall again and the risk for having another fall is higher. Studies have shown that one of the most important risk factors is a history of a previous fall. The staff should be eliciting information about previous falls and then altering the plan of care to take this higher risk for falls into account.

4. How did the fall occur? The circumstances of the fall and the risk factors have a huge impact on how you establish liability. The onus of responsibility rests with the healthcare provider, the licensed person and the facility.

Documentation of Falls

Let's assume the damages of a fall meet your threshold as a plaintiff attorney and you decide to bring the client in for an interview to obtain more information and to order medical records. Documentation is key. Typical investigation of the claim includes the questions below.

- What does the medical record say about the patient's risk factors for falls?
- What was the patient's mental state before the fall?
- Was the patient alert and oriented at the time of the fall?
- What did the nurse chart about how the fall occurred or how the patient was found?
- If the patient could speak after the fall, what did he or she say about the events leading up to the fall?
- Did the patient acknowledge a role in causing the fall? For example, in one particular circumstance a patient said to the nurse, "I know I should have used my call light to call for assistance." This is statement came from somebody who fell on her way to the bathroom and sustained a fracture. That nurse also contacted a nursing supervisor who wrote an additional note describing the status of the patient and what she had to say about her fall.
- Is the chart missing any description of the circumstances of the fracture? Did the healthcare provider fail to document this incident as a fall in the medical record because he or she considered it to be an "assisted to the ground" fall? Unexplained fractures or acute or chronic pain

localized to an extremity may indicate that a fall occurred. I recall one case in which the fractured femur eroded through the skin - there was no documentation of any injury. The failure to record a fall, even though perceived as non-harmful, provides the appearance of a cover up. This may be construed as tampering with the medical record, and significantly increases liability. Concealing the incident delays the diagnosis of injuries, prolongs pain and suffering, puts the patient at risk for dying for undiagnosed serious injuries, and puts the entire professional staff at a high risk for liability.

Work Up of the Case

The legal nurse consultant (LNC) assists the attorney by providing services to identify the liability, causation and damages associated with a falls claim. Some of the services may include those described below.

A chronology of medical care: the LNC goes through the records of the plaintiff from before and after the fall. The purpose of the review of prior medical care is to determine the baseline or condition of the patient before the fall.

- Was the patient prone to falls?
- Had the patient had a prior injurious fall?
- What were the risk factors that contributed to the fall? For example, a man who had a history of alcoholism tripped on a sidewalk. His blood alcohol was highly elevated when he went to the emergency department.

- Was the patient on any medications that could have caused dizziness?
- Are there any pertinent medical records that are missing?

The attorney uses the chronology to gain a full understanding of the patient's pre-existing conditions, injuries and the consequences of the fall.

A timeline: The LNC may prepare a brief outline of all of the significant treatment, including surgeries, hospitalizations, and outpatient treatment. The attorney uses this listing to prepare for depositions and to understand the scope of treatment.

A medical literature search: The LNC may be asked to look at how the literature supports or refutes the causation claims. Are the complications the patient developed after a fall those that could be attributed to the injury? For example, the patient claims she developed osteomyelitis after an ankle fracture. A patient with pre-existing back injuries claimed he developed herniated discs after falling on the ice on the post office steps.

A comprehensive summary of the medical records: The LNC, who becomes a testifying expert, prepares a detailed summary of the medical records, which explains the symptoms and treatment that resulted from the fall. This role is accepted under the Federal Rule of Evidence 1006, which permits a summary of voluminous medical records. The expert is not expressing opinions but is instead translating the medical records into understandable terms. More explanation of the role is provided in Patricia Iyer, Editor, *Medical Legal Aspects of Pain and Suffering,*

Lawyers and Judges Publishing Company, and Patricia Iyer, Barbara Levin, Kathleen Ashton and Victoria Powell (Editors), *Nursing Malpractice, Fourth Edition*, Lawyers and Judges Publishing Company. [2]

Location of expert witnesses: The LNC could be asked to locate experts to address specific points of a falls claim. The LNC may assist the attorney's analysis of a case in these types of situations, by finding

- a physician expert to provide an opinion that the mechanism of the fall was consistent with the injuries.
- a physician to determine if the patient's complications are plausibly related to the initial injury (this may be the same expert).
- a nursing expert to address the liability issue.
- a physician expert to determine if medical malpractice occurred after a fall that took place outside of a healthcare facility.

Identification of documents to be obtained during discovery: Using insider knowledge of the medical system, the LNC assists the attorney to determine which documents would be helpful for expert review of a case. The LNC identifies policies, for example, in a nursing malpractice case involving a fall. The LNC reviews the medical records supplied by the facilities and medical practices who treated the patient, and determines if the records are complete.

---

[2] Both texts are available at www.patyer.com.

Preparation for deposition and trial: The LNC prepares the attorney for deposition and trial by supplying updated chronologies and timelines, identifying key documents to be used as exhibits, educating the attorney in medical terminology, suggesting questions to ask the witness, and discussing strategy and trial themes. The LNC makes sure the attorney has a thorough understanding of the types of injuries falls may produce.

Discovery

These documents will aid in the analysis of liability in a malpractice case:

- Fall prevention protocols
- Policies and procedures for doing a falls risk assessment
- Instructions and policies for using bed alarms, chair alarms, wanderguards
- Policy for use of sitters
- Side rail use policy
- Incident reports
- Staffing records for date in question

Expert Witness Evaluation of Liability

Many states have regulations that govern who is qualified to act as a liability expert. A combination of recent or current clinical practice that matches the clinical setting where the fall occurred, excellent communication skills, and analytical ability, make a strong expert. Nursing experts should be evaluating the standard of care for nursing cases. [3]

---

[3] This subject is covered in more depth in Ray Fleming and Patricia Iyer, "Working with Nursing Expert Witnesses" in Patricia Iyer, Barbara Levin, Kathleen Ashton and Victoria Powell, *Nursing Malpractice, Fourth Edition*, 2011, available at www.patiyer.com.

There are so many factors that could cause a fall, but from a liability perspective, the issue that is of high concern for attorneys, risk managers, expert witnesses and insurance carriers is which of those falls could have been prevented. The questions below assume the fall occurred within a healthcare facility.

- Which falls should have been prevented by the actions of either the healthcare providers or the people who designed the environment in which the fall occurred?
- Was the patient identified as being at risk for falls?
- Were measures implemented to prevent the fall?
- Was the call light at the bedside utilized to call for assistance?
- Was the patient capable of using the call bell?
- Was the bed in its lowest position?
- Were lights on in the room or under the bed to help light the area at night?
- Was the patient appropriately monitored after the fall to detect injuries?
- Was the patient's risk for falls identified after the fall and the plan of care changed?
- Was the new plan implemented to minimize the opportunity for other falls to occur?
- Was the patient given anti-skid slippers?
- Is it possible to determine how soon the individual was found after he had sustained a fall?
- What was done at the time of the fall?
- What did the assessment reveal?
- Was there an injury?
- Did the nurse communicate the findings to the physician?

- Were X-rays ordered and performed?
- Was there an injury and how soon was that injury treated?
- If the patient fell and hit his head, was the chart reviewed, was the individual on anti-coagulation blood thinner such as Heparin or Coumadin?
- Was this communicated to the physician so that head scans could be performed to see if there was some type of bleed in the head?
- Was there a change in mental status after the fall?
- What were the vital signs?
- Were there specific conditions which contributed to the fall?
- Was the person assessed and monitored?
- What medications had the patient received prior to the fall?

Deviations

The plaintiff's expert witness may allege any of these deviations occurred. Below are some examples of deviations alleged in actual fall-related cases.

Failure to provide a safe environment

Nursing staff in healthcare settings may become the targets of a nursing malpractice case when injury results. The environment may have contributed to the fall by posing a challenge for a patient with a visual problem. A patient of any age may have difficulty seeing, but the issues are more common in the elderly. Nurses are expected to recognize the visual changes associated with aging and provide adaptive measures:

- use nightlights in the bathroom and bedroom
- avoid a cluttered environment

- avoid highly buffed floors that reflect overhead light with glare
- provide large print room door tags with the patient's name and room number
- use a high contrast color on the edges of steps
- keep clothes and objects in the patient's room in the same positions
- create lighting within the facility that is consistent, evenly distributed, and of adequate intensity
- place fluorescent or brightly colored tape around outlets, light switches, and doorknobs
- mark eyeglasses with the patient's name
- keep commonly used objects within reach of the patient so searching and stretching to reach something will not be needed

Failure to follow standards of care
- failure to follow the care plan intervention that two people were needed to transfer a patient
- failure to support a paraplegic patient during a shower caused a fall and fractured pelvis
- failure to respond to a patient's call for help resulted in the patient getting up on her own and falling
- failure to appropriately train staff in transfer techniques resulted in a head injury when the patient was being transferred out of bed
- failure to respond to a patient's request for help to get off a commode

Failure to use equipment in a responsible manner
- failure to use bed alarms and sensors

- failure to ensure that batteries were working in sensors
- failure to properly maintain a Hoyer lift, resulting in a fall
- failure to use a low bed
- failure to put up a side rail before rolling a patient on her side led to a fall off the bed
- failure to lock the wheels of a bed or wheelchair
- failure to ensure that doors to the outside or stairwells were not left propped open on units with cognitively impaired patients

Failure to communicate
- failure of the nurse to fill out forms instructing the aides on how to follow fall precautions for a woman with a previous history of a fractured hip
- failure to report a fall
- failure to instruct caregivers on proper transfer techniques

Failure to document
- failure to establish and record a plan to prevent falls in a patient with 57 falls and 18 head injuries
- failure to report and record details of a fall
- failure to record telephone orders for fall prevention measures

Failure to assess and monitor
- failure to monitor a patient who fell repeatedly, ultimately resulted in loss of an eye during a fall in a parking lot
- failure to assess and monitor a patient following a head injury led to undetected increases in intracranial pressure and death

Failure to act as a patient advocate

- failure to report signs of lethargy consistent with over-sedation, followed by a fall
- failure to question excessive doses of psychotropic medications
- failure to obtain medical examination after a fall

Healthcare providers are expected to act as patient advocates to secure help for their patients. A delay in treatment may occur because:

- The healthcare providers did not collect the appropriate data needed to assess the patient's condition. The person who fell was not thoroughly assessed and an injury was missed.

- The appropriate data was collected but the healthcare provider did not have the knowledge to critically analyze the data to find its meaning. The signs of a fracture were overlooked.

- The data was collected and analyzed, but the appropriate healthcare provider failed to respond to another person's concerns. The nurse could not get the attention of the physician or the nurse's concerns were dismissed.

- The concerns of the bedside clinician were heard, but the provider did not or could not make timely decisions about what to do about the changes in the patient's condition.

Falls Without Negligence

Healthcare providers used to believe that all patient falls were simply accidents and twenty years later we know that that's not true. Our knowledge is constantly changing and being updated. What we know now is that falls do occur by happenstance. We don't know why some patients fall and even though we've done all of the assessments, we've put into place interventions to help, they continue to still fall.

Defenses

Defense counsel and experts critically evaluate a falls claim to probe for weakness in the claim. There are several avenues of defense:

- **It did not happen here.** Check to see if it is possible the patient fell before entering the hospital or nursing home. Was pain in the injury site already present on admission? For example, a patient fell at a nursing home. The fracture was not detected, although he complained of pain. After he went to the hospital he fell again. Which fall caused the fractured hip?
- **The plaintiff is an unreliable witness.** The plaintiff attorney relies on the plaintiff's version of events, but the version cannot be substantiated and defies logic. The patient might be found on the floor, but cannot explain what happened due to delirium or dementia.
- **The nurse used nursing judgment.** The nurse assessed the patient before walking her to the bathroom and did not believe the patient needed a second person to assist. The nurse made a reasonable decision given the information available at the time. The nurse was not gifted with hindsight.
- **The patient was contributorily negligent.** The alert and oriented patient refused to follow instructions to call for help before getting out of

bed. Or the patient suddenly moved within the hydraulic lift sling and fell before anyone could reach her.

- **There are two schools of thought about how the events that led up to the injury should have been handled.** There is valid nursing literature to support how the nurse handled the situation.
- **There is no proximate cause between the fall and the injuries.** The patient may have fallen, but there were no injuries, or the patient's condition may have deteriorated for reasons other than the fall.
- **The plaintiff nursing expert did not define a particular deviation from the standard of care.** The expert's written report or testimony does not define specific deviations. The expert does not clearly define the standard of care, or offers a net opinion (not substantiated by references to the standard of care).
- **The plaintiff nursing expert referenced standards not in use at the time of the fall.** The expert might have cited standards published *after* the fall.

Key Points

1. Decisions about the statute of limitations, damages and liability govern which cases warrant closer investigation by plaintiff attorneys and their experts.
2. The medical record provides rich detail (or should) about the patient's condition before and after the fall.

3. Some falls are foreseeable and preventable with appropriate application of measures.
4. Deviations from the standard of care can be varied, individualized, and defined by a nursing expert.
5. Both plaintiff and defense attorneys should identify potential defenses.

The next section of the book focuses on another common allegation: failure to prevent pressure sores.

Pressure Sores

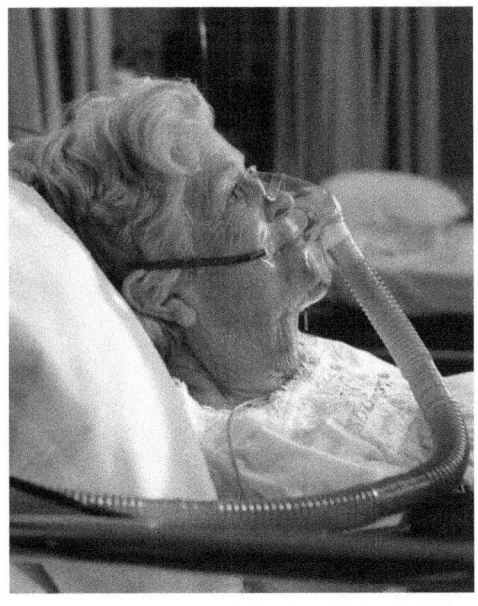

Chapter 5 Why Pressure Sores Happen

The first four chapters addressed falls as a common cause of lawsuits. Pressure sore cases are also common, potentially large damages cases. Like falls cases, pressure sore cases are often easy for a jury to understand. Most jurors have heard of bedsores and may believe that pressure sores are easily prevented by diligent medical care. Pressure sore cases, therefore, are potentially large verdict cases. The plaintiff may have graphic photos of large infected pressure sores. In making the argument that pressure sore development is a deviation from the standard of care, the plaintiff attorney may focus on the CMS position that Stage III and IV pressure sores are never events that should not happen in health care.

Pressure sores may develop in a patient who becomes debilitated as a result of surgery, trauma, illness or other causes. The second part of this book covers the topic in depth. Hospitals and nursing homes are the most common sites of debilitated patients, but pressure sores may develop wherever there are debilitated patients.

A pressure sore is a localized injury to the skin or underlying tissue, usually over a bony prominence, that is a result of pressure or of pressure combined with shear or friction. [4]

---

[4] Clinical Practice Guidelines for Pressure Ulcers, American Medical Directors Association.

Incidence

There is no central reporting agency that collects statistics on all pressure sores throughout health care. These numbers are estimates.

- There are 1.3-3 million sores in the U.S.
- The incidence in hospitalized patients is 5-10%.
- The incidence in nursing homes is 13%.
- The incidence in spinal cord injured patients is 39%.
- More than half of long term care patients with sores have methicillin resistant staphylococcus aureus (MRSA), a difficult-to-treat infection.

Federal and state organizations focus on regulations that are designed to reduce the incidence of pressure sores. Pressure sores are costly to treat, not only within hospitals and nursing homes but in the community after the patient is discharged.

Costs of Pressure Sores

In 2007, CMS stated that there were 257,412 pressure sore cases at a cost of $43,180/hospital stay for Medicare patients. Treatment of associated complications from a pressure sore may exceed $200,000 per patient, in addition to the costs of $20,000-$70,000 for wound treatment. The cost to treat pressure sores is $1.68 to $6.8 billion annually. For this reason, pressure sores are one of the conditions on the CMS list of nonreimburseable conditions, which affects reimbursement to hospitals. The government focused on the high cost of treating sores, which is at least 2.5 times the cost of preventing them. The cost of treating Stage IV sores is 10 times that of treating Stage II sores. (See below for definitions of stages of pressure sores.)

In many states, the state department of health also singles out prevention of pressure sores through regulations and making them reportable events. Requirements for reporting pressure sores vary from state to state.

Stages

Pressure sores develop from consistent pressure of soft tissue over a bony prominence of the body. The vast majority of them develop over the lower body (sacral area, hips, and feet). They are categorized by the depth of the wound, the layers and type of tissue that has been damaged. Here are terms used by many clinicians:

Deep tissue injury: The skin is purple or maroon skin, intact or has a blood-filled blister due to damage of underlying soft tissue.

Stage I: There is no opening in the skin, but a color change noted on the skin (red or darker), especially on that covering a bony prominence (heel, ankle, elbow, hip, sacrum, back of the head, around the ear). The darkness does not fade within 30 minutes of pressure being removed (non-blanchable). Sometimes there is also a change in the texture of the skin, from firm with resilience to mushy, boggy and painful to touch.

Stage II: The skin is open to a shallow depth, may drain a small amount of blood, or sero-sanguinous fluid (liquid that is blood tinged). It can be very painful.

Stage III: This is a wound that goes down through subcutaneous and fatty tissue but does not include muscle. This is a deeper sore than a Stage II. It may display tunneling (passages from the wound bed radiating outward toward healthy tissue). It can be extremely painful.

Stage IV: There is massive tissue destruction and drainage involved, can be deep and wide, and extend down to the bone. It is deeper than a Stage III. Surgery is frequently required to repair it.

Unstageable: There is full thickness tissue loss in which the actual depth of the sore is completely obscured by slough or eschar.

Note that the CMS guidelines deny reimbursement for the more serious pressure sores that develop in hospitals – Stage III and IV. Plaintiff attorneys most typically focus on these most serious and involved pressure sores.

Key Points

1. Pressure sores are costly.
2. Pressure sores are caused by unrelieved pressure.
3. Pressure sores are categorized in stages.

The next chapter addresses the damages aspects of pressure sores.

Chapter 6 Pressure Sore Injuries and Treatment

The pressure points, such as the heels, back of the head, and sacrum are common sites for sores. More than half of patients who develop a pressure sore while hospitalized will die within 12 months. It may take many months and even years for a pressure sore to heal. In the process, the patient may undergo extraordinary expense, inconvenience, flap surgeries, a colostomy to divert stool away from a sacral pressure sore, foot or leg amputations, and more. Potential complications of pressure sores include

- sepsis,
- osteomyelitis (bone infection),
- infectious arthritis,
- urethral fistulas (tunnels between the urethra and the vagina or bowel), and
- renal failure.

A few studies have been done to evaluate the impact on the quality of life of the patient with a pressure sore. The studies have revealed that pressure sores produce

- endless pain,
- restrict life activities, and
- a significant amount of coping on the part of the patient.

The endless pain is caused by the increase in discomfort that

- occurs as a result of moving, leading patients to

lay still,
- is associated with dressing changes and debridements (cutting off dead tissue), and
- is caused by alternating air mattresses.

Pressure sores may cause

- depression,
- feeling burdensome, powerless, or inadequate,
- worry, and
- wound odor that affects the patient and others.

Pressure sores can cause emotional distress in patients. A survey of patients with pressure sores showed that some patients believed healthcare professionals did not fully appreciate the pain of the sores and their complaints of pain were ignored. Patients may be too frightened to discuss pain with the doctor but may open up to a nurse, some other allied healthcare personnel, or a family member.

Treatment

Treatment of the pressure sore is dependent on the stage. The goal of treating Stage I sores is to prevent skin breakdown by relieving pressure and protecting the reddened skin. Once the top layer of skin is lost, the goals of sore dressings include keeping the sore bed moist, while keeping the surrounding skin dry, protecting the sore from contamination, and promoting healing.

The clinician has a variety of products to choose from for each stage of the sore. The factors to consider include the:

- sore characteristics (depth, condition of the surrounding skin, location near sources of contamination, presence and amount of drainage)
- impact on the patient (how many daily dressing changes are required)
- cost effectiveness of the product
- ease of use and cost of staff time to use the product
- safety, efficacy and likelihood of and potential severity of complications [5]

Most wounds can be treated with simple sharp removal of superficial nonviable tissue and infected tissue. Moist necrotic tissue is yellow or gray. Dry necrotic tissue is thick, hard, leathery and black. Just because a pressure sore has odor, and just because a pressure sore has drainage, doesn't mean it's infected. Culturing is not often done because it is so notoriously unreliable.

Wound VACS

Wound VACs are used to promote healing of a pressure sore. Over a million patients have been treated with negative pressure wound therapy since 1995 and it's gained international acceptance. There's an increasing evidence base for its use with over 300 peer reviewed articles.

Negative pressure wound therapy is a device that applies negative pressure, also defined as subatmospheric pressure. It's a suction pump that

---

[5] Clinical Practice Guidelines for Pressure Ulcers, American Medical Directors Association

delivers suction at 50-200 mm of mercury pressure, and it can be used for all kinds of wounds including pressure sores. The wounds do not even have to be technically open for this device to be used. Research on a cellular level shows it has significant impact in enhancing and improving wound healing as it

- removes wound drainage,
- decreases swelling by sucking the liquid from the wound,
- increases local perfusion,
- increases angiogenesis, which is new blood vessel formation, and
- promotes granulation tissue formation.

Usually the dressing change frequency can be every 48 hours. This reduces the pain associated with more frequent dressing changes. Clinicians often reserve the use of a VAC for big, serious wounds. VAC dressing changes may take between a half-an-hour to two hours. They are very time intensive.

There are serious contraindications found in the FDA monograph for the device. They include any exposed anastomosis where two sides have been sutured together, exposed vasculature, exposed nerve, or exposed organ. Placing a suction device over a vessel may cause the vessel to explode. The other issue has to do with the necrotic tissue. The VAC is a negative pressure, not a debridement device. (Debridement is the removal of dead tissue.) Wounds with necrotic tissue need to be debrided before they are appropriate candidates for negative pressure.

There are other clear risk factors that a reasonably prudent practitioner should seriously consider before ordering negative pressure wound therapy. A person is not a good candidate for a VAC device if there is a high risk for bleeding, receiving anticoagulants, has platelet aggravation factors or anything else that is going to cause bleeding.

Practitioners who order wound VAC therapy must follow the standards of care. Specific orders have to be written for each patient and wound that address the amount of millimeters of mercury used, how often the dressing should be changed, and with what materials. The standards of care come from the manufacturer's clinical guidelines. There are a number of internal consensus statements and reports, and the clinical literature. The ordering variables require some clinical judgment such as

- the amount of suction for a particular wound,
- whether that suction sucks continuously or on an intermittent pulse pattern,
- how often the dressings are actually done,
- the types and combinations of the foam or gauze, and
- knowing what contact layer should be used

These variables should be specified in the physician's order.   There are model order sheets available, but they are not universally used.

To have successful outcomes with negative pressure wound therapy, the facility has to have a trained inter-professional team that collaborates and communicates, and it's best that they be certified. The safety measures are important to incorporate and to ensure that all these things are documented, and that the checklists and order forms are used. And finally, there are wonderful educational materials for patients and caregivers that manufacturers have created that should be provided to patients and their caregivers.

Key Points

1. Pressure sores may cause prolonged suffering from pain and odor as well as limitations of mobility and socialization.
2. Pressure sore goals include keeping the sore bed moist and surrounding skin dry, protecting the sore from contamination and promoting healing.
3. Wound VACs may be useful for healing an involved pressure sore but carry risks for their use.

In the next chapter, you will learn how sores are prevented.

Chapter 7 Pressure Sore Prevention

Risk Assessment

The first step in preventing pressure sores is identifying the patient at risk. Facilities should use a standard, validated reassessment tool. There are two commonly used pressure sore risk scores: The Braden Scale and the Norton Scale. Each has different parameters and methods of scoring.

- **Braden Scale** - Sensory perception, moisture, activity, immobility, nutrition and shear.
- **Norton Scale** - Physical condition, mental condition, activity, mobility and incontinence.

These are the subscales of each tool. A recent systematic review of risk assessment scales found that the Braden Scale had the optimal validation and best sensitivity/specificity balance when compared to the Norton Scale. The Braden Scale has demonstrated a high degree of interrator reliability for registered nurses but unacceptably low interrator reliability for nursing assistants and licensed practical nurses. (Interrator reliability refers to whether two people using the same tool would come up with the same score for the patient.)

The Braden scale is the most widely used tool in the U.S. It is easy to use, has been clinically validated, and requires minimal training. It addresses many of the issues that can affect the risk of pressure sores. Keep in mind that the Braden scale will not capture all of the risk factors that can contribute to the development of pressure sores. A thorough patient history is important to ascertain such contributing factors as age, medications, and medical conditions, including a history of pressure sores. Many risk factors for pressure sore development have been identified; however, a hierarchy of risk factors has not been determined. More than 100 risk factors of pressure sores have been identified in the literature.

Factors include

- diabetes,
- multiple sclerosis,
- peripheral vascular disease,
- renal disease,
- obesity,
- cerebral vascular accident,
- sepsis,
- hypotension,
- age 70 or older,
- current smoking history,
- dry skin,
- being on steroids (which affect wound healing),
- history of a Stage III or IV pressure sore,
- low or high body mass index,
- impaired nutrition or malnutrition,
- impaired mobility,
- altered mental status,
- urinary and fecal incontinence,
- physical restraints,
- patient refusal of some aspects of care and treatment
- cognitive impairment, and
- malignancy.

Completion of the risk assessment is not enough. Dr. Braden herself has said on many occasions, "It's not just about the score. It's what you do with the score." Did the patient's score deteriorate? If incontinence becomes an issue was there evidence that the staff implemented an incontinence guideline? If the skin breakdown got worse, did the staff change the plan of care to add a skin barrier?

CMS recommends that nurses consider all risk factors independent of the scores obtained on any validated pressure sore prediction scales because all factors are not found on any one tool. Whatever tool is used, successful healthcare users of the tool characteristically have:

- Administrative level and nursing staff buy-in and support.
- Development of an actual process integrating the pressure sore risk reports into ongoing quality improvement processes.
- Facility champions to keep the effort focused and on track.

Every patient with limited mobility is at risk for developing a sacral, ischial, trochanteric or heel sore. Daily assessment will rapidly identify patients with beginning sores. A full evaluation of a sore is mandatory. A simple recording of measurements is minimally acceptable.

Any break in the skin must be documented and quickly treated. It is essential for staff to regularly monitor pressure sores at consistent intervals to make sure treatment is working. Effective wound beds are free of scar tissue and infection. A moist wound healing environment facilitates granulation tissue formation.

In addition to protecting healthy skin from damage, good nutritional status is important for effective wound healing. The healthcare team should evaluate the patient's nutritional status. The albumin and prealbumin levels measure nutritional status. One of the easiest ways to do this, other than looking at the current weight compared to the ideal body weight, is to look at protein levels.

Albumin measures protein levels. Albumin has a long half-life, about 20 days. Because of its half-life, this makes albumin a *late* index of malnutrition.

Prealbumin is another protein indicator; it is different from albumin because it has a shorter half-life. This makes it a more sensitive protein indicator at 2 days half-life. Prealbumin must be screened for all patients, especially those who have wounds because it is the best monitoring index for one's nutritional status. Its shorter half-life makes it possible to evaluate one's nutritional status in a shorter timeframe since prealbumin levels can be obtained from the patient 1-2 times a week. [6]

Pressure should be relieved from the wound and other high risk areas. Cellulitis (reddened inflamed tissue) is treated with antibiotics, moist dressings and surgery. Drainage is a potential sign of infection and must be eliminated.

Several key recommendations to minimize the occurrence of pressure sores are:

---

[6]   http://www.differencebetween.net/object/comparisons-of-food-items/difference-between-albumin-and-prealbumin/

- Avoid using hot water when washing the skin.
- Use only mild cleansing agents.
- Avoid low humidity because it promotes scaling and dryness.
- Minimize friction. Do not massage reddened areas over bony prominences.
- Provide frequent turning and repositioning with a turning schedule that is based on the patient's individual risk factors.
- Minimize pressure through support surfaces.
- Inspect skin during bathing and turning.
- Evaluate and manage fecal and urinary incontinence. Do not allow the patient to sit in waste for prolonged periods.
- Being on a pressure-redistributing mattress or cushion does not negate the need for turning and repositioning.
- Maintain adequate nutrition and hydration.
- Do not drag the patient up in bed, which causes shearing of the sacral tissues. Many hospitals are now utilizing an overhead lift system which helps to move the patient in the bed as well, which helps decrease the amount of back injuries that nurses may sustain during their work day.
- Use lotions and creams to protect the skin from incontinence.
- Help postoperative patients out of bed as soon as practicable to prevent immobility and pressure sores.
- Elevate heels off of the mattress to prevent pressure.

Although preventing pressure sores is a multidisciplinary responsibility, nurses play a major role. Studies have suggested that pressure sore development can be directly affected by the number of registered nurses involved and time spent at the bedside. A growing level of evidence suggests pressure sore prevention can be effective in all healthcare settings. Prevention needs to be viewed as more than just the care of the skin. It should encompass patient education using multiple forms of education in a variety of languages, clinician and administrative staff training to understand responsibilities for preventing and treating pressure sores, development or refinement of toolkits and protocols and documentation.

Biological therapies, such as growth factors, have been shown to promote wound healing. Physical therapy is important for all immobile patients.

Key Ingredients of Prevention
The NOULCERS bundle developed by the New Jersey Hospital Association reduced pressure sore incidence by 70 percent and pressure sore prevalence by 30 percent in 20 months across care settings.

- **N**utrition and fluid status
- **O**bservation of skin
- **U**p and walking or turn and position
- **L**ift (don't drag) skin
- **C**lean skin and continence care
- **E**levate heels
- **R**isk assessment
- **S**upport surfaces for pressure redistribution

Institute for Healthcare Improvement Guidelines
These are the key ingredients of the IHI Guidelines:

1. Conduct a pressure sore admission assessment for all patients.
2. Reassess risk for all patients daily.
3. Inspect skin daily.
4. Manage moisture.
5. Optimize nutrition and hydration.
6. Minimize pressure.

Key Points

1. It takes a multidisciplinary team to identify risk factors and implement a plan of care to prevent pressure sores.
2. Risk assessment, skin protection, nutritional management, and pressure minimization are essential ingredients of a prevention plan.
3. It is not enough to complete risk assessment tools. The healthcare team must take action when they recognize a patient at risk.

The next chapter addresses how to analyze the liability associated with a pressure sore case.

Chapter 8 Liability for Pressure Sores

Analysis of a Pressure Sore Case

Again, I'd like you to envision sitting in a plaintiff's law firm. The phone rings and the voice at the other end of the lines says, "My mother was in the hospital and developed a large pressure sore on her backside." What are some of the questions that you should be asking the caller? Aside from the questions that help you determine the statute of limitations, the questions that elicit clinical details should help you gather as much information as possible about the circumstances of the pressure sore.

- Why was the patient in the hospital?
- How old was she?
- What was her physical condition before the sore began?

The complexity of pressure sore cases is affected by other illnesses, such as infection, circulation, diabetes, Alzheimer's, and the end of life. Evaluation of the full medical record is needed to obtain more details about the pressure sore and the patient's condition.

Work Up of the Case

The legal nurse consultant (LNC) assists the attorney by providing services to identify the liability, causation and damages associated with a pressure sore claim. Some of the services may include those described below.

A chronology of medical care: The LNC goes through the records of the plaintiff from before and after the pressure sore development. The purpose of the review of prior medical care is to determine the baseline or condition of the patient before the pressure sore development.

- Was the patient prone to pressure sores? Once the skin is damaged by a pressure sore, leaving scar tissue, it is at higher risk for future breakdown.
- What were the risk factors that contributed to the pressure sore development? For example, did the patient have other sores on her body? Was she immobile, incontinent, and poorly nourished?
- Are there any pertinent medical records that are missing?

The attorney uses the chronology to gain a full understanding of the patient's pre-existing conditions, injuries and the consequences of the pressure sore.

A timeline: The LNC may prepare a brief outline of all of the significant treatment, including surgeries, hospitalizations, and outpatient treatment related to the pressure sore. The LNC details the development and progression of the sore, indicating the dimensions and descriptions. I have worked on cases involving patients who developed more than one sore, and have prepared timelines that tracked each one. The attorney uses the timeline to prepare for depositions and to understand the scope of treatment.

Analysis of the origin of the sore: The LNC may be asked to look at the medical records and photographs to help determine if the sore is likely to be due to pressure or to another origin. For example, there are several non-pressure related causes of skin breakdown:

- The wound may be a foot sore related to peripheral neuropathy in a diabetic. The patient may have small or large blood vessel disease if his diabetes is chronic and not well controlled.
- The patient may have reduced blood flow to the legs from diabetes, coronary artery disease, elevated blood lipids or peripheral arterial disease. This may affect the toes as an ischemic sore (one due to a loss of blood supply).
- The patient may have a venous foot sore from venous insufficiency or following phlebitis.

A comprehensive summary of the medical records: As described in Chapter 4, the LNC, who becomes a testifying expert, prepares a detailed summary of the medical records, which explains the symptoms and treatment that resulted from the pressure sore. This is particularly effective if the patient was alert, oriented, and able to experience the discomfort associated with a pressure sore.

Location of expert witnesses: The LNC could be asked to locate experts to address specific points of a pressure sore claim. The LNC may assist the attorney's analysis of a case in these types of situations, by finding

- a physician expert to provide an opinion on the origin of the pressure sore – a vascular surgeon, geriatrician, wound care specialist or internist may be appropriate.
- a wound care expert physician to determine if the medical care was within the standard of care.

- a nursing expert to address the liability issue.
- a nursing wound care expert to evaluate the wound care.

Identification of documents to be obtained during discovery: Using insider knowledge of the medical system, the LNC assists the attorney to determine which documents would be helpful for expert review of a case. Key documents often include the pressure sore risk assessment policy, pressure sore prevention policy, and pressure sore treatment procedures. The LNC reviews the documents supplied by the facilities and medical practices which treated the patient, and determines if the records are complete.

Preparation for deposition and trial: The LNC prepares the attorney for deposition and trial by supplying updated chronologies and timelines, identifying key documents to be used as exhibits, educating the attorney in medical terminology, suggesting questions to ask the witness, and discussing strategy and trial themes. The LNC makes sure the attorney has a thorough understanding of the stages and treatment of pressure sores. The LNC may be involved in the preparation of demonstrative evidence. The attorney may want to use illustrations of the stages of pressure sores. The LNC assisting the plaintiff attorney may sift through photographs of the pressure sore to select those that have the highest impact.

Key Elements of Pressure Sore Analysis
The high stakes aspects of pressure sore cases makes it important for the attorney, risk manager, expert witnesses and legal nurse consultants involved in

a case to consider key elements. The following section of the chapter provides a roadmap for analysis.

What Was It?

Is the wound truly a pressure sore, or could it be a failed surgical wound, incontinence associated dermatitis, or a venous or arterial ulcer that resulted from poor circulation? Did the patient undergo a Doppler arterial study to determine if the sore was caused by vascular insufficiency or by pressure? Was the wound a chronic one that was present before admission to the facility? Was it a chronic one being managed at home? Did the wound represent skin changes at life's end when all body systems were breaking down?

Where Was the Sore on the Patient?

Sores on the feet or toes may be related to vascular insufficiency. As noted above, there are several non-pressure related causes of skin breakdown. I know a very good plaintiff nursing home attorney, meaning he handles nursing home cases, who will not litigate any case involving heel sores. He will only take sacral pressure sores because he doesn't want to get into the battleground of vascular insufficiency, arterial insufficiency, and the causation of foot sores. Sores on the back of the head, elbows, sacrum, and hips are much more likely related to pressure.

Are There Pictures?

Healthcare providers are not required to take pictures of pressure sores, but many do to permit comparison of the sore over time. Pictures in the medical record are usually in color. The attorney may request color copies of those pages. Healthcare staff should obtain good quality pictures. They should take the pictures at a consistent distance from the body, not modify a digital image, and include the patient's name, date, and sore location within the image. Family members may take pictures with lesser quality cameras, but these may be the only ones available. Pictures of deep pressure sores may have a huge impact on a jury.

Family or facility photographs are usually admitted into evidence, although they have been fought about and challenged. The facility's photos are often clearer than those taken by the family using cell phones. The clearer photos may help the facility defend itself. On the other hand some families are sophisticated, use high quality digital cameras, and document the entire progression of the pressure sore. It would be difficult for a facility to prevent family members from taking pictures. That would raise questions about what the facility was trying to hide.

What Year Did the Pressure Sore Develop?

What federal and state regulations were in place? If the sore occurred in a hospital, what The Joint Commission and state regulations affected the delivery of care and prevention of pressure sores? If the sore developed after 2004 in a nursing home, the nursing home F-Tag 314 was in effect. This standard states,

"Based on the comprehensive assessment of a resident, the facility must ensure that—
1.   A resident who enters the facility without pressure sores does not develop pressure sores unless the individual's clinical condition
2.   demonstrates that they were unavoidable; and
3.   A resident having pressure sores receives necessary treatment and services to promote

4.   healing, prevent infection and prevent new sores from developing".

In 2007, the National Pressure Ulcer Advisory Panel's definitions of a deep tissue injury or an unstageable sore were introduced in the academic community, but they didn't actually come into clinical use until later, depending on the setting. Deep tissue injuries existed before the terminology changed. But the clinical staff cannot be held accountable for not using the term "deep tissue injury" before the introduction of that term. Previously, the term "Stage 1" was used. There was no other language for that condition.

Where Was the Patient Before the Pressure Sore Was Discovered?

Deep tissue injuries may result after a patient fell at home, for example, and was lying on the floor, undiscovered, for several hours or days. Was the patient on a back board in the emergency department for a prolonged period? Was the patient on an insufficiently padded operating room table on her back for a long surgery? Look for the clues in the medical record.

Who Is the Appropriate Expert to Retain?

Do you need both a nursing and a physician expert witness? A *nurse* evaluates the way the nurses did or did not follow the standard of care. A *physician* evaluates the physician management of the patient, and the causation between the sore and the ultimate medical condition or demise of the patient.

A *vascular surgeon* addresses the causation question when the pressure sore could be related to vascular insufficiency. A *dietician* may be needed if the facility's dietician did not provide oversight of the patient's nutritional status. A *wound care nurse* reviews the performance of the wound care nurse at the facility.

There are two certifications for wound care nurses: WOCN and CWCN. The WOCN is granted by the Wound Ostomy and Continence Nurses Society at http://www.wocn.org/. The CWCN is a Certified Wound Care Nurse. The certification is granted by the organization for Wound Care Nurses at www.woundcarenurses.org.

How Often Did the Nurses Assess Skin Integrity?
Were risk assessments and preventive measures consistently used? Evidence-based research recommends assessment intervals for various care settings as follows:

- Acute care patients in the ICU should be reassessed daily with unstable patients being reassessed every shift.

- Medical surgical and other patients should be assessed at least every 24 hours. Many facilities do this more often because patient status can change rapidly. The Institute for Healthcare Improvement recommends daily assessment.

- Long term care patients should be assessed on admission, then reassessed every 48 hours for the first week. They should be reassessed weekly for the first month, and monthly to quarterly thereafter or then whenever health status changes. Bergstrom and Braden found in their long term care research that 80% of pressure sores developed within two weeks of admission. Ninety-five percent developed within three weeks of admission. Quarterly risk assessment tools are clearly too infrequently done.

- Home health care patients should be reassessed at every visit. Family members should be shown how to perform skin assessments.

- What did the facility state was the appropriate interval for assessments? Did the staff follow their own policy?

- Did the staff take action at an early point in the development of the pressure sore? Did they notify the physician of the early signs of skin breakdown? Did they develop a wound care plan of care?

Was There Clear Accountability For Assessments?

There should be clear expectations of staff conducting the risk assessment, which include which nurse is responsible for the first assessment and for subsequent assessments. This should be defined as to who and which shift is responsible for doing the assessment.

A full skin assessment should be done on admission so that the staff detects pressure sores that have developed elsewhere. The chart should document their descriptions. The staff must document in detail about a pressure sore, including dimensions and stages.

In 2008, the CMS "Present on Admission (POA) Rule" was introduced. This regulation states that a hospitalized patient's skin must be assessed within a narrow window of time after hospital admission defined as "by midnight the next day" with no provision for weekends or holidays. Under the CMS guidelines, pre-existing sores present on admission must be documented by the attending physician or CMS-defined provider. The facility is not denied reimbursement for Stage III or IV pressure sores that were present on admission. Pressure sore prevention protocols, once formulated for the patient, must be documented. Without proper documentation, a tremendous legal and financial burden shifts to the provider.

Following is a summary of the general POA reporting requirements:

- The POA indicator is required for all claims involving Medicare inpatient admissions.

- POA is defined as present at the time the order for inpatient admission occurs.

- A POA indicator is assigned to principal and secondary diagnoses.

- Issues related to inconsistent, missing, conflicting, or unclear documentation must be resolved by the provider.

- If a condition would not be coded and reported based on Uniform Hospital Discharge Data Set definitions and current official coding guidelines, then the POA indicator is not reported.

- CMS does not require a POA indicator for the external cause of injury code unless it is reported as "other diagnosis." [7]

Did Staff Carry Out Preventative Measures?
Staff should be aware of and follow the protocol for pressure sore prevention in high risk patients. The procedures should conform to best practices and avoid incorporating the interventions which have been proven to be harmful such as massaging bony prominences, and using donuts under the sacrum, and sheepskins.

What Is the Quality of the Documentation?
Is the case about documentation or is it about the practice? What did the staff do? What does the record show was done? Is the charting markedly incomplete or too perfect looking? I have seen wound care charting that was so perfectly done because the nursing staff sat down and created one year of charting at once. They failed to recognize they documented the interdisciplinary team met on a major holiday when most of the staff were not in the building. I taught a program in 2012 with two plaintiff and one defense attorney in which we talked about medical records. The plaintiff nursing home attorney said that in 50% of the cases that he litigates the aides were charting care when the resident was not in the building. That's an issue that's very easy for juries to understand. It may not have been related to the core issues in the case, but it inflames the jury and the plaintiff attorneys get great leverage from that type of charting practice.

---

[7] Carol A. Armenti, "Preventing Healthcare-Acquired Conditions Means Never Having to Say You're Sorry", in Patricia Iyer, Barbara Levin, Kathleen Ashton and Victoria Powell (Editors), Nursing Malpractice, Fourth Edition, available at www.patiyer.com.

Does the chart contain a description of:

- Location, size, and color of the wound
- Amount and type of exudate
- Odor
- Nature and frequency of pain
- Color and type of tissue and character of the wound bed, including evidence of healing or necrosis
- Description of wound edges
- Stage

These are the types of descriptions that are typically charted. Universal wound care terminology must be consistently used. The documents should be reasonably consistent with one another. Risk assessment forms and skin wound sheets, and treatment administration records should be reasonably complete and consistent with each other.

Minor discrepancies between how the staff were staging a pressure sore sometimes occur. These are staging issues; they're not quality of care issues. Staff needs to carefully document the condition of the skin on admission to a hospital or nursing home, and on transfer or discharge.

Analysis of liability involves the tricky issue of following protocols for turning. Did the aides follow the turning schedule? How did they document compliance? How much detail did they provide? How often was the patient moved for other reasons? Go through a record and figure out how many times a person sat up in bed, went to therapy, was cleaned up for incontinence, or had her bed changed. Most people are being moved more than every 2 hours.

Was There a Plan of Care?
Did the nurses formulate and implement plans of care? Did they recognize the patient as being at risk for skin breakdown? Were the plans consistent with the standard of care? Were preventative measures in place? What kind of mattress was under the patient? What product did the staff put on when they realized the person had a wound? It is difficult to defend a case when there was no documentation that there was a wound care plan of care implemented when the wound was first recognized.

The standard of care now requires that every wound patient's wound plan of care is individualized. It's also considered essential that a wound care team approach needs to be used. If there was a plan of care, was it consistent with the overall plan of care?

If the wound changed and deteriorated, is there correlation between the nursing notes, the physician progress notes and the orders? If the wound was getting worse, there should be nursing and physician observations about the wound, changes in the plan of care, involvement of the dietician, and appropriate consults. How were the nurses dealing with the corrosive effects of incontinence? Was the obese patient on a special bariatric bed? Was the patient on a pressure relieving mattress? How long did it take for the facility to obtain the special mattress once the need was recognized?

The case may rest on the details of the nursing documentation regarding frequency of turning, amount of diet eaten, etc. These indicate whether the plan of care was consistently followed. As the expert looks at the chart, those are important ways he or she makes the decision about whether the standard of care was met. The challenge is to paint a picture that laypeople are going to be able to understand in a courtroom about the overall plan of care.

In facilities that have not yet adopted electronic medical records there is much duplication of documentation. Staffing cutbacks may have set up the nursing staff for failure. Many are unable to meet the documentation requirements of some of these facilities. The facilities must take a serious look at how they can simplify things even if it's still on paper so that people just document the essential things.

For example , is it realistic for aides to chart that they turned patients every two hours? If they have 10-15 patients to care for, it is more realistic for them to chart they turned the patient every 2 hours during the shift rather than to document every turn.

Did the Plan of Care Address Pressure Redistribution, Topical Treatments, and Nutritional Support?

Were these needs addressed in a timely manner? Were the interventions consistent with the standard of care? Were the interventions based on sound clinical protocols and evidenced based practice? For example, was Silvadene ordered twice a day instead of once a day, and used as a topical antibiotic? There are lots of appropriate dressings for a particular wound. It is inaccurate for an expert to provide an opinion that says, "The only dressing that would've worked on this patient is this..." For any given wound there are probably 3 or 4 dressings that would be appropriate choices. Some may be better than others, but again the judgment is whether it meets the standard of care.

Was There Good Communication?

If a person had a pressure sore for 4 months and it was never mentioned in the physician's progress notes that's a problem with communication. Did the doctor respond to calls the nurses made about skin changes? If the responses were not appropriate, did the nursing staff go up the chain of command? Did they act as advocates for the patient by getting the appropriate level of expertise? If they worked in a long term care facility, for example, where there was no wound expert, what was their obligation to get an appropriate wound consult or send somebody to a wound center? If they were in a remote area without a wound center, how did they get that person to the appropriate level of expertise?

If no healing was occurring, did the nurses consult with the physician or enterostomal therapist? Did they get an expert consultation? The plan should be updated as the wound or skin condition changes.

Studies have shown that if a wound with the ability to heal is not 30% smaller at week 4, despite optimal local wound care, it is unlikely to heal by week 12. Advanced therapies should be considered. If a wound is unlikely to heal because of inadequate vasculature or coexisting illness, advanced therapies are seldom indicated and their chance of success is minimal. Stage I and II pressure sores, when treated appropriately, need not deteriorate if there is adequate, proper and timely preventive measures and treatment.

Was There Adequate Institutional Support?

Institutional support involves providing staff and supplies, and supporting the importance of pressure sore prevention. For example, a nursing home resident went to a wound care center, which provided a set of recommendations for treatment. The nursing home did not follow them because of the cost associated with the product that was recommended by the wound care center. This is part of the challenge of trying to deliver care across the continuum of care and dealing with limitations on treatment availability in one setting versus another setting. What a wound center may prescribe and what a long-term care facility or homecare agency can provide may be totally different. These factors influence analysis of liability.

The institution supports quality improvement and educational activities needed to focus on pressure sore prevention and treatment. The administration assures that the results of studies are shared with the staff so that they may be involved in developing goals for the reduction of sores. Staff needs to know how to activate the involvement of the wound care nurse, if such a person is on staff, and if a consult is needed.

The staff should be educated to prepare an individualized care plan with specific interventions designed to prevent and treat pressure sores. The plan should be consistent with the patient's overall plan of care. The plan needs to be documented and communicated clearly and in a timely manner to the patient, family, and/or healthcare power of attorney and relevant members of the patient's healthcare team.

There should be a permanent method of denoting a patient at risk for pressure sore development and means of communicating that risk status to all who care for the patient.

Did the Physician fulfill His or Her Responsibilities?

The physician should examine the patient from head to toe, front to back. Too often only the front of the body is seen. Part of the physician's responsibility is to identify risk factors for a patient developing a pressure sore, and to review records and talk to the patient about a previous history of pressure sores. The physician assesses the patient's overall physical, psychosocial health, nutritional health, and current medical conditions. He or she looks at the presence of contractures, dementia, depression, and terminal illness.

Once a pressure sore has developed, the physician also should review nursing documentation to monitor the effectiveness of treatment, as well as examining the wound. The physician identifies factors that affect the pressure sore healing and acts to modify those factors, if possible. He or she should order vascular studies to rule out severe peripheral vascular disease as a cause of heel pressure sores, monitor lab values, such as albumin, and weights, for evidence of malnutrition.

Defenses

As discussed, pressure sore cases can be challenging for the defense team. The damages are obvious, and the liability may be easy to establish. The defense team has some potential avenues for its defense of the claim.

The Pressure Sore was Unavoidable

This is a potent battleground between expert witnesses. The definitions stated in the CMS Guidance Document for Surveyors apply to long term care facilities:

Avoidable – the nursing home resident developed a pressure sore and the facility did not do one or more of the following:

- Evaluate the resident's clinical condition and pressure sore risk factors
- Define and implement interventions that are consistent with resident needs, resident goals and recognized standards of practice
- Monitor and evaluate the impact of the interventions
- Revise the interventions as appropriate

The definition of an unavoidable pressure sore is closely patterned on the factors that CMS defined as within the control of the nursing home.

Unavoidable – the nursing home resident developed a pressure sore even though the facility had

- Evaluated the resident's clinical condition and pressure sore risk factors
- Defined and implemented interventions that were consistent with resident needs, goals and recognized standards of practice
- Monitored and evaluated the impact of the interventions
- Revised the approaches as appropriate

The patient who develops pressure sores is often sick with multiple medical problems. These conditions may exist, which make it difficult to prevent or heal pressure sores:

- Extremely thin body
- Widespread cancer
- Several failing organs
- Severe blood vessel disease
- Terminal illness

No studies have found that prevention of all pressure sores is possible. Significant reductions in the incidence of pressure sores are possible.

The defense team may have to argue that maybe the care wasn't perfect, but would it have made a difference in the end? In so many of these cases the patient may have been on the best support surface. He could have had all the nutrition pumped into him by tube feeding, but none of that would have been absorbed. He would have ended up with tube feeding diarrhea. He was at the end of his life and going to breakdown no matter what anybody knew how to do. There is limited understanding of how to intervene to prevent pressures sores in terminally ill patients.

The Sore had an Arterial or Vascular Origin
Foot sores cases are often easier to defend than sacral pressure sore cases. A foot sore, as previously described, may be due to an underlying diagnosis of arterial or venous insufficiency. What are the other comorbidities? Is the patient diabetic? How long has the patient had diabetes? Is there micro-vasculature and macro-vasculature compromise and neuropathy?

There is usually more than just one diagnosis. Were wound workups done? Were options given?

The Sore was Present on Admission; it Developed Elsewhere

Careful analysis of the medical record may show that the patient entered the facility with a pressure sore that developed elsewhere. Documentation of the skin condition may be found in the hospital emergency department records, the nursing admission assessment and the physician history and physical. Documentation of the skin condition of a nursing home resident may be found in the facility's admission assessment, the minimum data set, and the physician history and physical. The defense strategy may be to shift the blame to the facility that sent the patient into the facility with a pressure sore.

The Patient Was Uncooperative

An alert, oriented patient has the right to refuse preventive care. A mentally competent person who does not want to turn or reposition or be cooperative with the care needed to prevent pressure sores poses a challenge for the medical team. It is difficult to perform positioning on a patient who is resistant. A person with enough mobility placed on her side may easily flip onto her back. A patient may refuse clearly needed care to pressure points and sores. The healthcare team, when confronted with such a situation, needs to investigate the causes of the patient's behavior and work towards a plan that addresses the underlying reasons for the refusal. If all efforts fail, ultimately a competent person may refuse to cooperate and develop pressure sores.

Sources of Pressure Sore Standards of Care

American Medical Directors Association, Pressure Ulcer Clinical Practice Guideline 2008, www.amda.com

EPUAP/NPUAP International Pressure Ulcer Clinical Practice Guidelines, 2009

World Union of Wound Healing Societies, Best Practices Documents and Woundpedia, www.wuwhs.org

Wound Ostomy Continence Nurses Society (WOCN) Pressure Ulcer Guideline 2010, www.wocn.org

There is a document called The Long-Term Care Enforcement Procedures which comes from AHCA and there is a phone number and a website. This is the document that's used by surveyors and it has the F-Tags in it. It used to be a watermelon pink color, so nursing home attorneys refer to it as the watermelon book even though it's no longer watermelon color. If you're going to be involved in doing nursing home cases, that is an important document to have in your possession. You can get information about this at AHCAPublications.org. Their phone number is (800) 321-0343.

Key Points

1. A systematic evaluation of the variables that affect liability helps the attorney, legal nurse consultant and experts evaluate a pressure sore case.
2. Wounds on the feet may have a vascular origin unrelated to pressure. A physician expert will

help the legal team identify the pressure versus vascular foot sores.

3.   Pressure sore cases are high risk for the defense but viable defenses exist.

The last section of this book addresses risks associated with intravenous therapy.

Intravenous Related Injuries

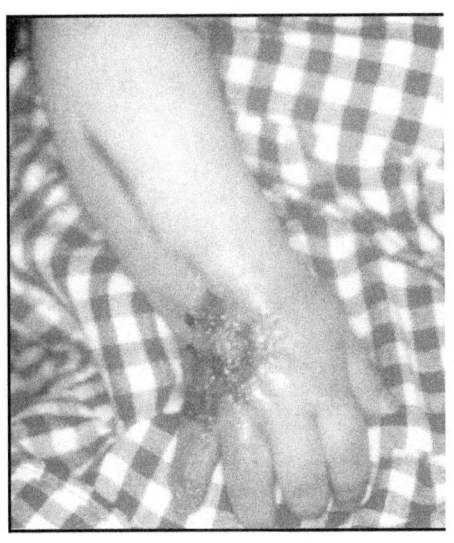

Chapter 9 Why Infiltration and Extravasation Happen

Almost every patient who is admitted to a hospital has some kind of IV therapy. The last section of the book focuses on complications of IV therapy: infiltration, extravasation, catheter and air embolism and infection. Although medical technology has become more sophisticated, the risks and serious outcomes of this type of therapy remain present. They can be as minor as a small area of fluid under the tissues (infiltration) or as serious as death from air introduced into the blood (air embolism).

Definitions

It's quite difficult to make medical personnel as well as attorneys, and legal nurse consultants understand the difference between infiltration and extravasation. A *vesicant* is a drug that is capable of causing severe tissue damage. *Infiltration* is by definition the accidental infusion of a *non-vesicant* solution into the tissue. An *extravasation* (pronounced ex-*trav*-a-sa shun) is an accidental infusion of a *vesicant* solution into the tissue. The vesicant is typically a caustic medication or a concentrated intravenous solution.

High Risk Patients

Certain patients are at high risk for damage if caustic medication gets into their tissues. Neonates and children, by virtue of having small veins, are at particularly high risk. The cover page of this section and the next picture show damage caused by extravasation of medication.

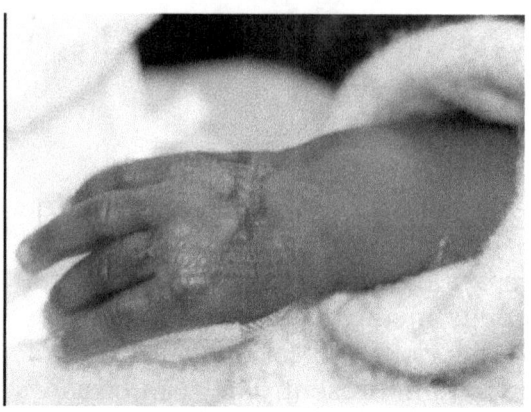 In neonatal units, premature infants almost always get concentrated sugar solution and almost all of them have calcium or potassium in them. These are just three of the commonly used caustic medications that are infused into the tiny veins of an infant or child. It is within the standard of care to use a foot vein, but nurses should avoid inserting intravenous needles into the veins of the ankle because when babies move their feet, the catheter can come out of the vein. This is one way the caustic medications can enter the tissues.

The elderly are also at higher risk for skin damage because their veins are weaker. As part of the aging process, the outer wall of the vein becomes transparent. This makes the elder's veins fragile and very prone to infiltration and extravasation.

The critically ill patient who is dependent on caustic medications such as Dopamine or Levophed to maintain blood pressure, is also at high risk for extravasation.

Chapter 10 Injuries and Treatment: Infiltration and Extravasation

Consequences of Infiltration

Many infiltrations that are quickly detected resolve without treatment. The attorney is most likely to become involved in litigation when an infiltration results in significant injuries. The infiltration of intravenous fluid can lead to an accumulation of a large amount of fluid under the tissues. Intravenous pumps will continue to pump fluid into the tissues even if the catheter moves out of the vein. When there is no more space left in the tissue, finally the pump will alarm to signify there is an occlusion and the pump will shut down. The tissues can absorb hundreds of mls/ccs of fluid in the tissue before the pump actually alarms. The fluid compresses the other structures in the tissue such as the nerves, resulting in numbness and tingling within the swollen area.

A large infiltration may result in a serious complication of compartment syndrome. Nurses are expected to know the symptoms of compartment syndrome and identify patients at risk for its development. The assessment of pulses, sensation, and movement of a limb will detect early signs of compartment syndrome. This is a dreaded complication that can cause massive damage to a limb. The syndrome develops because the fascia that surrounds the compartment does not stretch when swelling occurs. The swelling causes increased pressure on the structures in the area and thus blocks blood flow and impairs nerve function.

Compartment syndrome is a painful condition that involves increased pressure in a muscle compartment. The pressure escalates to dangerous levels and compresses muscles, nerves and blood vessels. This can cause tissue death if not detected or acted upon in time. The sooner the surgeon takes action the better. Early intervention in compartment syndrome will relieve the pressure on the nerves and hopefully save the function of the nerves. Acute compartment syndrome is a medical emergency that develops over hours.

The nursing standard of care requires the nurses to detect the symptoms and get a physician to examine the patient. The patient must get into the operating room as soon as possible for a fasciotomy. The surgeon makes multiple incisions in the arm to relieve the pressure. The fluid almost shoots out of the tissue because it is under such pressure. The patient can be left with enormous scarring. Compartment syndrome can cause permanent nerve injury to the arm. These patients can be left with complex regional pain syndrome and possibly a lifetime injury of nerve compression.

Consequences of Extravasation

Extravasation of caustic medications can cause tissue death. The vesicant causes extreme pain, irritation, blisters, and redness. Many chemotherapeutic drugs, such as Adriamycin, are caustic. Electrolytes are probably the most caustic medications that healthcare providers infuse. These drugs include potassium chloride, calcium chloride, and calcium gluconate. Any type of calcium is very caustic to the tissue. Some other caustic drugs are Dopamine, Levophed, Thyroxine, and Sodium Bicarbonate; those are just a few. Intravenous antibiotics are not caustic. They can cause irritation to the vein, but they tend not to cause tissue necrosis or tissue gangrene.

Extravasation is a risk associated with giving vesicants. Sometimes the risk is due to the concentration of the medication and the solution. Giving a concentrated potassium chloride solution increases the amount of tissue damage that can be caused if it gets into the tissue. A drug that has a very high risk of and potential for tissue necrosis should be given through a central venous catheter that has been inserted into a large blood vessel, such as the superior vena cava in the upper chest. The next picture shows a chemotherapy extravasation that occurred when the drug leaked out of a port implanted in the patient's chest.

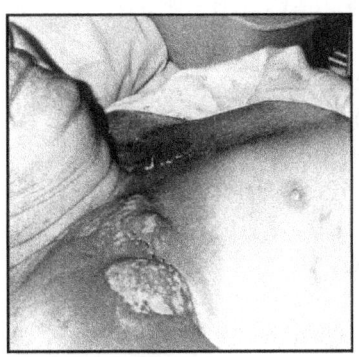

Some of these drugs spread in the tissue by attaching to the fat molecules. The injury may be first noted as local pain. It may progress into blisters, and then tissue sloughing (pronounced as *sluffing*) or loss. An extravasation that starts in a hand may progress up into the arm. That's why sometimes surgeons have to amputate the arm, to stop the spread of that extravasation all the way up the arm. There can be tendon damage, muscle damage, nerve damage and skin loss. Neonates may require an amputation right above their ankles if the extravasation destroys the joint. Consider the significant damages of losing a foot or a hand. These cases can be very difficult to defend.

The next picture shows a patient's arm after chemotherapy extravasation. The arm was amputated.

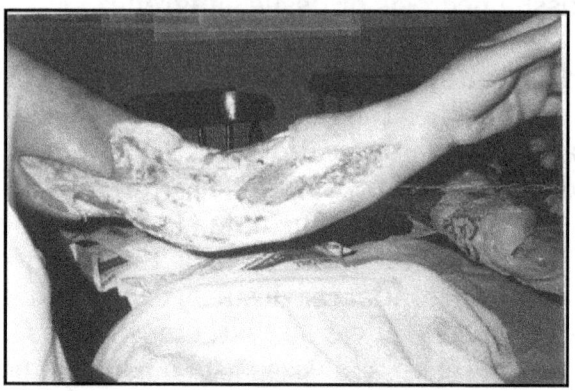

Treatment of Infiltrations and Extravasations

It used to be common to apply warm or hot compresses to the tissues of an arm with infiltrated fluid containing a medication. Medical professionals should now know a warm compress may worsen the situation because it may cause the drug to crystallize in the tissue. Some medical professionals treat infiltrations with ice; others elevate the extremity. There is no scientific data to support the application of compresses, and there is a study that shows that elevation of the arm really can be more painful than non-painful. The trend now is to not do anything for an infiltration but observation. Nurses are expected to monitor the site for color changes and temperature changes.

Treatment of extravasation is also controversial. There are antidotes for some caustic medications, but not all. Some healthcare providers order heat; some people use cold; others use sodium sulfate for some chemotherapeutic drugs. There is little evidence that any of those treatments work to help decrease the symptoms of the extravasation or the progression of the extravasation. Prevention is the best practice because once the vesicants get into the tissue there is very little medical professionals can do to stop the injury. There will be damage if the patient has a large amount of that vesicant in the drugs making contact with a large amount of tissue.

Chapter 11 Prevention and Early Detection of Infiltration and Extravasation

As you have seen from the previous chapter, significant damages can result from in infiltration or extravasation. The analysis of these cases often centers around the standard of care for preventing these outcomes. The analysis of liability is often not clear cut, in part because the standard of care may not be well delineated. For example, consider the phrase "frequent monitoring of an intravenous site." What is the definition of frequent monitoring? A facility's policy may not provide a specific time frame.

Many hospital policies state the site should only be checked once a shift. The definition of a shift may have changed from what used to be an 8-hour shift to a 12-hour shift. What length shift does the facility's policy refer to? Does the nurse recognize that the frequency of site checks should increase if the patient is receiving a caustic medication? If the nurse administers potassium chloride for a four-hour infusion and only checks the site at the beginning and at the end of the infusion, the patient could sustain significant damage if the whole infusion went into the tissue.

Assessment of an intravenous site is the responsibility of registered nurses. A hospital that reduces the number of registered nurses, which increases the number of patients the registered nurse is assigned to, contributes to the risks of infiltration and extravasation. It is very difficult for the registered nurses to take care of a large number of patients. Even though it takes seconds to assess an intravenous site, a nurse may be tied up with responsibilities that interfere with site assessment. A devastating injury can occur if an infiltration or extravasation is not detected for six to eight hours.

Please note that this section of the book refers to the *nursing* standard of care. This does not mean that other healthcare professionals are not also involved in checking intravenous sites. For example, an anesthesiologist monitors an intravenous site during an operation, as do rescue squad members who start IVs and give fluids. Early detection of infiltration or extravasation is certainly the responsibility of any medical professional who administers intravenous fluids.

Early Signs

Prevention of infiltration and extravasation depends on early detection of the same symptom: swelling. Picture the IV catheter or the plastic tube sitting in the vein. For infiltration or extravasation to occur, the needle must slip out of the vein. Now it's punctured a hole in the vein and the medication is now going into the surrounding tissue. Obviously the main thing the nursing staff will see is immediate swelling. The intravenous fluid will collect under the tissue and it will get bigger and bigger and bigger as the amount of fluid inside the tissue increases.

In addition to assessing for swelling, the nursing standard of care requires checking for coolness at the site. The nurse has to touch around the IV catheter to check the temperature of the skin around the IV site. If the IV fluid goes into tissue, the site will be cool to the touch because the IV fluids that were infusing are not body temperature. Therefore, the two main symptoms medical professionals should look for are swelling and coolness.

Both infiltration and extravasation begin with swelling and coolness. Suppose an attorney asks a defendant nurse, "How can you tell the difference between an infiltration and extravasation if you're looking for only coolness and swelling?" The answer should be, "It depends on what the nurse is infusing. The nurse has to recognize whether the solution contains a vesicant (caustic medication) because that increases the risks.

Chapter 12 Liability for Infiltration and Extravasation

Once again, I'd like you to envision sitting in a plaintiff's law firm. The phone rings and the voice at the other end of the lines says, "My mother was in the hospital. Her arm swelled up from an infiltration. Do I have a case?"

What are some of the questions that you should be asking the caller? Aside from the questions that help you determine the statute of limitations, the questions that elicit clinical details should help you gather as much information as possible about the circumstances of the infiltration.

- Why was the patient in the hospital?
- How old was she?
- What was her physical condition?
- What was done to her arm after it became swollen?
- Did she require surgery to reduce the swelling?
- What does her arm look like now?
- Does she have any impairment of her ability to use her arm?
- Did she have any physical therapy after this occurred?
- Has she been diagnosed with a chronic pain syndrome?

Infiltration Damages and Liability

Med League occasionally gets calls from attorneys looking for expert witnesses to review cases about infiltrations that have occurred in the hospital without leaving any permanent damages. The calls are few in number because plaintiff attorneys are aware that there are no damages from a small infiltration. The problem is time limited and self-correcting - the tissue absorbs the extra fluid. However, large infiltrations that result in significant damage may be caused by a delay in detection of the tissue changes.

The fact that an infiltration occurred does not necessarily indicate there was a deviation from the standard of care. Healthcare professionals cannot prevent all infiltrations from occurring, even with the best nursing care and the best patients. The catheter can still move out of the vein and cause fluid to go into the tissue. Patients' veins become fragile and the longer the admission and more frequent requirement for restarting the intravenous, the greater the risk of infiltrations. For this reason, healthcare professionals may insert a peripherally inserted central catheter (PICC) which is typically threaded up the arm to a point near the heart. This catheter may stay in for much longer periods than intravenous catheters inserted into veins in the lower arm. (Healthcare professionals need to undergo special training in order to insert PICC lines. The correct placement of the line is checked with radiological studies before the line is used.)

Extravasation Damages and Liability

Damage from extravasations relates to the amount of fluid in the tissue. A small amount of a vesicant solution under the tissue may result in a little skin blister. It will heal on its own, and may not even result in a scar. There is not going to be enough fluid in the tissue to cause any significant damage to the surrounding structures. However, the calls that Med

League gets about extravasation injuries are typically about a large amount of damage with significant blistering and skin sloughing. The analysis of liability focuses on the frequency of monitoring and the timeliness of detection of abnormal signs.

Work Up of the Case

The legal nurse consultant (LNC) assists the attorney by providing services to identify the liability, causation and damages associated with infiltration and extravasation claims. Some of the services may include those described below.

A chronology of medical care: The LNC goes through the records of the plaintiff. The LNC will look at the site checks that were documented and the documentation that describes the evolution of the injury and treatment.

A timeline: The LNC may prepare a timeline that may be an abbreviated version of the chronology. The attorney uses the timeline to prepare for depositions and to understand the scope of treatment.

A comprehensive summary of the medical records: As described in Chapter 4, the LNC, who becomes a testifying expert, prepares a detailed summary of the medical records, which explains the symptoms and treatment that resulted from the infiltration or extravasation.

Location of expert witnesses: The LNC could be asked to locate experts to address specific points of an infiltration or extravasation. The LNC may assist the attorney's analysis of a case in these types of situations, by finding

- a surgeon to describe the surgical treatment needed to address compartment syndrome.
- a neurologist to explain the nerve damage from compression.
- a nursing expert to address the liability issue.

Identification of documents to be obtained during discovery: The LNC assists the attorney to determine which documents would be helpful for expert review of a case. Key documents often include the procedure for insertion of IV needles, the policy for monitoring intravenous sites, and the protocol for treatment of infiltration and extravasation. The LNC reviews the documents supplied by the facilities and medical practices who treated the patient, and determines if the records are complete.

Preparation for deposition and trial: The LNC prepares the attorney for deposition and trial by supplying updated chronologies and timelines, identifying key documents to be used as exhibits, educating the attorney in medical terminology, suggesting questions to ask the witness, and discussing strategy and trial themes. The LNC makes sure the attorney has a thorough understanding of the standard of care and damages associated with infiltration and extravasation. The LNC may be involved in the preparation of demonstrative evidence. The plaintiff attorney may want to use illustrations of the anatomy of the nerves, and scars left by a fasciotomy. Family members, healthcare providers or professional photographers may be able to supply photographs of the scars.

Medical Record Documentation

Assessment of an intravenous site for signs of infiltration or extravasation is a nursing function. As such, the results of that assessment should be documented either in a handwritten flow sheet or electronic medical record. The documentation must reflect what actually occurred, rather than a perfunctory or rote charting. It is all too easy for nurses to copy and paste the electronic documentation from a prior shift without verifying all of the information. It is also easy for nurses to become "click happy" – checking off items in the electronic medical record without verifying the accuracy of each item. A nurse who documented she checked the IV site every 2 hours would have difficulty explaining why a huge infiltration resulted, one that would have evolved over several hours.

Vague documentation complicates analysis of liability. The term, "IV infiltrated" is an example. What does that mean?

- Was the patient having any complaints?
- What was the drug that was in the tissue?
- When was the infiltration discovered in relationship to the beginning of the nurse's shift?

Rather than properly document the size of swelling, it is commonplace for nurses to refer to an area as small, moderate or large. These are subjective terms that are open to interpretation or questioning during a deposition. The standard of care requires a nurse who detects swelling around the IV site to measure it. A 5-centimeter area of infiltration is small. A 10 x 15 centimeter area is huge and would imply that the nurse was not properly checking the patient and missed the signs.

A pattern that I have seen is that the next nurse coming on the shift seems to be the one who typically finds the swelling as opposed to the one who was on the prior shift. That leaves questions about how long the swelling was undetected. In an extravasation case, the next nurse may be the person who finds blisters. The extremity turns purple and is painful to the touch. This type of scenario requires attorneys and expert witnesses to backtrack through the documentation to figure out:

- When was the IV site last checked?
- What was the condition of the site at the time of the last check?
- In the event of an extravasation, what medication was given?
- What time was it given?
- Who gave the medication?
- When was the physician notified of the changes in the site, particularly if a large infiltration, signs of compartment syndrome, or extravasation occurred?

All these questions help legal professionals figure out when the injury actually occurred. It may take a little bit of detective work to find that out. The main focus is determining when the healthcare professionals documented the site assessment or the early symptoms of infiltration and extravasation - swelling and coolness to the touch. The blisters of an extravasation occur in hours or days and may progress to deep tissue injuries. The most serious cases involve fasciotomy, debridements or amputations. Look for consultations to the plastic surgery service or the hand service or orthopedic service. Those requests trigger that something serious occurred.

Discovery

The attorney who is either defending a case of this nature or is considering taking it on as a plaintiff case is going to want to know some more information other than the medical records of the individual. The facility should supply the nursing policies and procedures specific to IV care. Also, obtain the orientation program description used for the training of the nurses when they hire them, which should include validation of competency. The hospital has the duty to provide a qualified nurse to take care of the patients. The attorney should also ask for the Joint Commission reports and should check the Joint Commission website for additional information about the facility's accreditation status.

These documents will aid in the analysis of liability:

- Incident report
- Policy on IV site monitoring
- Procedure for treatment of infiltration or extravasation

Liability Expert Witness Evaluation of Standards of Care

Nursing expert witnesses with experience in administering intravenous medications and observing intravenous sites are the ideal candidates to evaluate the standards of care in an infiltration or an extravasation case. There are certain standards of care that experts may refer to that provide some guidance on what should have been done.

The Oncology Nurse Society (ONS) has vascular access device guidelines and chemotherapy recommendations for practice. They are very broad; they may not form definitive statements. Additionally, they are only recommendations or guidelines.

The Infusion Nurse Society (INS) has standards of practice which are published every few years.

The Association of Vascular Access (AVA) does not provide standards; they do write position papers.

Many infusion (administration of intravenous fluids) standards are not evidence-based. They are not written based on basic research because there is an absence of such research for infusion therapy and vascular access (inserting needles into veins) methods. Many of the practices are rooted in tradition instead of research. While the standards exist, they vary from broad to specific.

Deviations
The plaintiff's nursing expert may identify some of these specific deviations.

Failure to follow standards of care
- failure to monitor the IV site
- failure to respond to a patient's request for help when she noticed her arm becoming swollen
- failure to respond to a patient's complaint of local pain or burning at the IV site
- failure to recognize the patient as being at high risk for an IV therapy complication
- failure to monitor motor and sensory function in a patient at risk for compartment syndrome

Failure to use equipment in a responsible manner
- failure to respond to IV pump alarms
- failure to keep the IV pump alarm on
- failure to use a transparent dressing so an IV site could be monitored
- failure to verify the intravenous needle was in the vein before administering a caustic medication
- failure to select a proper site for an IV needle

Failure to communicate
- failure of the nurse to communicate critical signs of a developing IV therapy complication

Failure to document
- failure to document the condition of the IV site
- failure to record the size of an infiltration
- failure to record the size of the intravenous needle that is in place

Failure to timely obtain treatment after the IV therapy complication
- Failure to obtain prompt physician evaluation of an large infiltration, compartment syndrome or extravasation

Defenses
- **The nurse used nursing judgment.** The patient had very poor veins; the nurse used the best location available.
- **We saved the patient's life.** The patient was very ill; infiltration and extravasation are known risks of using IV fluids/medications.
- **There are two schools of thought about**

how the extravasation should have been treated. There is valid medical literature to support how the complication was treated.

- **The nurse recognized the symptoms of compartment syndrome from infiltration but there was no surgeon/operating room available.**
- **The plaintiff nursing expert did not define a particular deviation from the standard of care.** The expert's written report or testimony did not define specific deviations. The expert did not clearly define the standard of care, or offered a net opinion (not substantiated by references to the standard of care).
- **The plaintiff nursing expert referenced standards not in use at the time of the intravenous therapy.** The expert might have cited standards published *after* the patient was treated.

Key Points

1. Infiltrations and extravasations injuries are not always preventable.
2. The amount of fluid in the tissue affects the damages. If there's a small amount of fluid in the tissue the damages are limited. If the staff was monitoring the patient carefully, they caught it early, and the patient will probably have zero injury.
3. A large amount of swelling, either from an infiltration or extravasation, causes injuries. That's when patients can get permanent injuries.

The next chapter focuses on another type of intravenous injury: nerve damage from direct contact with the nerve.

Chapter 13 Why Nerve Injuries from Venipuncture Happen

Whenever a healthcare provider sticks a needle through the skin in search of a vein there is a risk of injury. Needles may be inserted to start intravenous fluids or medications, or to obtain blood. Nerve injuries from an intravenous needle insertion are common allegations. The most common medical complaint is that as soon as the needle is inserted the patient feels an immediate, sudden electric shock sensation going down his arm. Some patients say their fingers will feel a jolt or the fingers shoot out involuntarily. Picture a needle going into your arm and making contact with the nerve. It's not a burning pain; it's not a throbbing pain; it's not even excruciating. It's a sudden and unexpected shock-like sensation going down the arm. That's the classic symptom of nerve contact.

Confirmation of Nerve Injury

Nerve injury cases are very difficult cases from the plaintiff position. The patients are often written off as malingers because if you look at their arms, there might not be anything that looks different. There are no markings on the arm; there are no changes in the arm. Their two arms may look basically the same, so people don't see any outward injuries such as an extravasation where there is a big chemical burn. It becomes very difficult to prove to a jury that there was in fact nerve injury and the patient is really hurting. I've worked on some of those cases of people who have these kinds of damages and it is a nightmare for them. It may be hard to convince a jury that person is really suffering. They're difficult cases that may result in large medical damages such as a nonfunctional extremity.

A neurologist is typically involved in the patient's care to help to determine the etiology of the symptoms. The neurologist will sometimes order nerve conduction studies or EMGs (electromyelography) for muscle studies. Usually these tests are done together; nerve conduction studies will show the velocity and the amplitude of the nerve conduction. But a patient may have an injured nerve and the nerve conduction study can be normal. That makes it very difficult to rely on these tests. Most patients don't even agree to have the EMG done because the tester has to stick lots of needles into the muscles of the arm and it's very painful. But just because there is a negative nerve conduction study doesn't mean that the patient doesn't have an injury. But if there is a positive nerve conduction study, you can be sure the patient has a serious injury.

Treatment

Patients may sustain significant injuries to the nerves; they may develop a little scarring on the outside of the nerves - a neuroma. Many patients have conservative therapy first - physical therapy, pain medications. They may progress to stellate ganglion blocks on their necks which are extremely painful. They need to have a huge series of injections: 12-16 of these injections to their neck. Typically they get very short-term relief from their pain, but the procedure is so painful that over time most people won't agree to continue with it because they don't get enough relief from the pain.

Sometimes these patients will have surgery on the nerve; sometimes they will ask to have the nerve surgically removed. The nerve can be actually severed in the arm. The surgeon drills a hole into the bone in the arm and implants the nerve into the bone. Another option is a nerve transplant. The neuromas are visible during surgery. The surgeon may take a photograph, which may be used as demonstrative evidence.

None of these treatments is particularly successful. Many patients end up on long term pain relievers, which have very unpleasant side effects. A lot of patients start out on these drugs but don't usually stay on them very long.

Many patients suffer horribly because the problem with this nerve injury is that it may become progressive as complex regional pain syndrome. Patients may suffer a nerve injury in the wrist, but symptoms may travel up their arm and into their chest, into their other arm and down into their legs over time, and there's nothing to stop the spread of this. The injury may result in terrible, debilitating pain. Most patients don't even leave their home because the pain in their arm is so significant.

Chapter 14 Prevention and Liability Analysis of Nerve Injuries

The previous chapter explained that there is little that can be done to treat a severe nerve injury. Prevention becomes essential. A variety of healthcare providers start IVs or remove blood for testing:

- Phlebotomists
- Rescue squad workers
- Physicians
- Nurses

The essential components of prevention are the same regardless of who is inserting a needle into a vein. Anyone who is inserting an IV or drawing blood is responsible for knowing the anatomy of the arm and the hand. The healthcare provider needs to know where the veins, arteries, and superficial nerves are located. That is the biggest issue for every court case - identifying veins. Attorneys commonly use an illustration of the anatomy of the arm and ask the defendant (or expert witness) to identify the structures in your arm. No matter who the provider is - a technician, a nurse, a doctor - he or she is responsible for knowing the anatomy. Not everybody's anatomy is the same but the provider has to know where the same basic structures and high risk areas are for a nerve injury.

High Risk Areas

The first of the areas where the nerves are at high risk for contact is the inner aspect of the wrist right above the palm. The radial nerve is extremely superficial in this area right above the thumb on the very low part of your wrist. People who are inserting IVs or drawing blood should never use this place. It is too high risk. The radial nerve and the median nerve are very superficial in these areas.

Some people say, "I put IVs there all the time, I haven't hit a nerve." But it only takes one time, and if the provider knows the nerve is superficial there is no good reason to use this site. The provider should place three fingers on the crease of the wrist, and avoid starting an IV in the area covered by the fingers. Even though this is a high risk area, it is commonly used and also commonly associated with nerve injuries. The reason why a provider is tempted to use this area is that he or she can see the vein. But that does not justify its use.

The second of these two areas is the inner part of the elbow (antecubital area, pronounced *an* - tee - cu-bit-al). It has very big structures. This is the primary place where healthcare providers draw blood. The needles are short – they are inserted and removed. But they're not supposed to be used for IVs because that involves a longer catheter. It's meant to stay in place for a couple days. The median nerve is extremely large there; the brachial artery is extremely superficial there, so there is an increased opportunity for hitting the nerve or artery. Also, if the patient gets an infiltration, if the needle moves, it travels through the vein and goes into the tissue. There's a little recessed area in your elbow - you can feel it. It's very hard to detect infiltrations until they're pretty advanced.

Staff in the radiology area commonly use the antecubital site for injecting intravenous dye or contrast. This is not recommended because they hook the needle up to a power injector and they inject the fluid in seconds. They could inject a 100 ml (a little more than 3 ounces) of fluids in about two seconds. This could put enormous pressure on the vein and cause lots of damage in that elbow area.

When I review rescue squad records, I commonly see the squad members use the antecubital site for IV insertion. They think it's an easy vein to use because they can see it. The most important thing is to feel the vein, not to be able to see the vein. But those veins are very short in the antecubital area. The patient is moving his elbow all the time. That tends to cause high risks for infiltration. The Infusion Nurse Society standards state providers should not insert IVs into areas of joint flexion, including the wrist and the elbow, because the movement increases the risk of the catheters puncturing the veins. If you can picture the catheter, it almost acts like a piston inside the vein and it can wear a hole in the vein causing the fluid to go into the tissue. Intravenous needles inserted by rescue squad members may be assumed to have been inserted in less than ideal (dirty) situations, and are often removed once the patient is in the emergency department.

The femoral area (in the groin) is an undesirable site for long-term access. The Centers for Disease Control, the Food and Drug Administration, and The Joint Commission all say the femoral vein is the worst site healthcare providers could possibly use. It is hard to keep it clean; it's hard to put a dressing on it; it's hard to keep it secured. The infection rate in these femoral lines is somewhere between 20-40%.

But healthcare providers like to use femoral veins because they are easy to get to and they can put them in pretty quickly. But for routine therapy, this is not an ideal site. This is just not acceptable because of the infection.

Inserting intravenous lines into the jugular veins is becoming more common. There's a big effort for nurses to be putting in jugular PICC lines. A PICC line is a Peripherally Inserted Central Catheter. It's about 25 inches long. It typically starts in the vein in the arm above the elbow and goes all the way through the big vein in the center of your chest - the superior vena cava. A long-term catheter can be in for months.

Several states, such as Pennsylvania and California, have approved nurses inserting jugular IVs. Nurses are being trained so that if they can't get a PICC line in someone's upper arm, they should be able to do that in jugular sites. There is a big increase in the amount of jugular lines being placed now. The jugular vein is a high risk blood vessel because it is close to the big carotid arteries in the neck. When providers insert the needle into the carotid artery by mistake, they may infuse fluids into the brain and the patient dies. There is also a huge vagus nerve in the neck. The proximity of these structures results in a serious opportunity for a serious life threatening complications.

Early Detection of Nerve Injury
Early detection plays a role in recognizing the symptoms associated with the nerve injury. Whoever is putting in the needle - whether it's for drawing blood or starting an IV - is responsible for recognizing the symptom of nerve contact. The symptom would be electroshock sensation or numbness and tingling radiating up and down the arm, involuntary extension of somebody's fingers; again, not necessarily

excruciating pain, but sudden unexpected shock-like sensation. Consider the fact that many people who are inserting IVs don't know nerve anatomy and certainly don't know the symptoms associated with nerve contact. When the patient says, "Oh, my gosh I feel an electric shock sensation going down my arm," the response of the clinician may be, "That's normal. I just put in a needle in your arm." But that's not normal.

Liability Analysis and Expert Witness Questioning

The patient will have some pain on insertion of a needle. The key points are:

- The healthcare provider should use an appropriate site for insertion of the needle.
- The provider should confirm he or she has correctly placed the needle in the vein before proceeding.
- The provider should immediate stop if the patient complains of an electric shock sensation.

At deposition or trial, the attorney questioning an expert witness about this point may ask what kind of pain would be normal. The pain of the needle going through the skin should be minimal. It should not be prolonged or shock-like or extensive or excruciatingly painful. Anything like that is a sign that something is wrong. It is up to the clinician or the technician who is inserting the device to recognize the symptom.

The attorney questioning an expert witness may ask, "Can you prevent all nerve injuries?" Many healthcare providers assert that this is not possible. There are times when the high risk areas have to be used. The provider may accidentally hit some nerve, and can't exactly tell before he gets started where the nerve is going to be. That's why he has to know the symptoms of nerve contact so he can recognize if he has hit the nerve. The chance of hitting a nerve is minimized if the provider uses a very shallow angle or tilts the needle to minimize the opportunity of hitting the nerve - not going too deep and not going too far.

If the needle makes contact with the nerve and the patient says, "I have an electric shock sensation going down my arm," the correct intervention is then to immediately remove the device. If the provider hits the outside of the nerve, then a little scar tissue (a neuroma) will form at the point of contact. The patient can still have complaints of numbness and tingling in her arm upwards of a year. It may take 12-18 months for that injury to go away.

A credible expert should testify that the provider may insert a device with the right technique in the right areas, and make contact with the nerve. If the provider takes the needle out, the injury that results may be just a neuroma on the nerve which resolves in a year. But avoidance of high risk sites reduces the risk of nerve injury. Additionally, patients may testify that, "The nurse came in and inserted an IV in my wrist. As soon as she did that, I felt an electric shock sensation. I told her and she said 'That's normal', and then she pushed the needle in a little further." This is a classic description from patients with these injuries. The needle was on the nerve. The second push results in piercing the body of the nerve. Now the fibers of the nerve have been cut or severed. This may become a permanent, progressive painful lifetime injury, and there is no treatment for that injury. A credible expert should testify that it is negligence to proceed with the IV insertion after a patient reports the electric shock sensation.

The most common defense of these cases is to assert that even with the best technique, it is possible to injure a nerve. The patient may move her arm; the anatomy may be unusual. Additionally, the defense may challenge a diagnosis of complex regional pain syndrome by having the patient examined by a defense medical examiner to dispute the presence of the syndrome.

Key Points

1. Healthcare providers should avoid inserting intravenous needles in the high risk areas of the inner wrist and inner elbow area.
2. Injuries to these patients are devastating.
3. Serious adverse complications of nerve injuries are preventable with proper care. When patients have significant nerve injury or have permanent nerve injury, these are all the result of deviations from the standard of care. That does not happen unless providers weren't doing their job; they weren't caring for the patient properly.

The next chapter addresses rare but potentially fatal complications of intravenous therapy: catheter and air embolism.

Chapter 15 IV Catheter Embolism and Air Embolism: Causes and Treatment

Catheter Embolism

A catheter embolism occurs when a piece of IV catheter tubing breaks off and starts traveling in the blood. There are two main types of catheters: short ones that are inserted into a hand or arm, and central catheters that are inserted into the upper arm or one of the large veins, such as the jugular vein or subclavian vein (in the upper chest). The little IV catheters that healthcare providers put in the arm or hand are short; they're about an inch and a quarter. It is rare for short ones to break off. If a small fragment of that breaks off, it probably lodges somewhere and gets walled off and doesn't really cause any harm to the patient.

The real risk occurs when patients have central lines. When the catheter is removed, a piece may break off. The catheter may snap and break. Perhaps 6-8 inches of the catheter may float into the patient's body, and that is significant. The standard of care requires the person removing a central catheter, particularly a peripherally inserted central catheter, to measure the catheter on removal and record the inches in the patient record. The provider needs to know the length of the catheter at the time of its insertion in order to detect a shorter catheter coming out of the body. The provider should inspect the catheter and look for any signs of breakage.

If the nurse is the person removing the catheter and finds out through measurement that there is a missing piece, the next step is to immediately notify the physician. When a piece breaks off and the healthcare provider is aware of the breakage, it is possible to attempt to retrieve the catheter. The physician will probably send the patient to interventional radiology to visualize the catheter fragment. The piece most often becomes lodged in the pulmonary artery. The providers have to get the piece out because it will cause a clot to form. Under fluoroscopy, they'll put the wires in to retrieve it and pull it out through the femoral vein. The wire is like a lasso; it's a wire with a loop on the end. Under fluoroscopy, they can see the image and they go in and they lasso it - put the loop around the catheter fragment, tighten the lasso and then pull it out.

Removal of a piece of catheter is usually successful if the problem is detected early. If the healthcare provider can get it in the first couple days, it's great. But if they find it later, it can have serious consequences. A piece may become embedded in an organ and necessitate removal of the organ. If the catheter piece lodges in the pulmonary artery, it narrows the flow of blood from the artery. The blood doesn't get through the body as quickly as it needs to; this can become life threatening.

Air Embolism

Air embolism is defined as simply the presence of air in the vascular system, in the venous system or the arterial system. It can cause anoxic encephalopathy as well, which is the lack of blood supply to the brain due to presence of air in the blood system. It is an air bubble or a block of air that is floating through the venous system which displaces the blood and therefore blocks blood supply to that area.

Air embolism represents a serious adverse event. The Centers for Medicare and Medicaid Services (CMS) have defined it as one of the never events. CMS and many private payors do not pay for the treatment of a hospital acquired air embolism. Treating an air embolism costs close to $66,000 per patient admission.

Air embolism from central venous catheters is on the increase. Death is the outcome of a significant size air embolism. Jugular lines are now on the increase; they are very high risk for air embolism - during the maintenance of the lines and also during the insertions. The serious nature of air emboli (plural of embolism) is worsened by the fact that healthcare providers receive very little training about how to prevent and detect the emboli.

The first central venous catheter was developed in 1967 and that's when health care first started to see the real serious issues related to air embolism. It's very rare to have air embolism in a peripheral line, so when these central lines became more prevalent, then air embolism became a bigger issue.

Risk Factors
Several types of patients are at risk for air embolism. Air embolism may develop in a surgical patient. Even in neurological surgery when the patient is upright, the surgeon has to be very careful because air embolism is a real risk in those procedures. Any kind of head and neck surgery is also very high risk for air embolism.

Air may enter the venous system through

- a catheter that has a hole in it,

- a cap that comes off a catheter,
- a catheter that has been disconnected from the IV tubing,
- during removal of the catheter, or
- manual injection of air into a catheter.

Patients with central lines are at high risk for air embolism. They have large lumen tubes that rest close to the heart. Peripherally inserted central lines are also at high risk. There are four elements that have to occur in order for air embolism to occur.

1. There has to be an opening right into the venous system. Putting on the wrong kind of dressing over an IV insertion site can be deadly. Just putting a band-aid over it or a piece of gauze and tape is incorrect. That's certainly not an air-occlusive dressing. The patient could cough, sneeze or hiccup, suck air right through the dressing and be dead in seconds.

2. There needs to be the right amount of air. Most experts readily agree that when there is more than 30 ccs (an ounce) of air in at one time, that's enough to cause damage to the patient. Air has to be pumped into or injected into a peripheral IV catheter. In one case, a radiologist was doing a venogram (injection of dye) on a patient. He used a 30 ml syringe and forgot to put the contrast in. He injected over 30 ml of air in seconds into the patient and that was enough to kill her. An air embolism can occur if the IV tubing is not primed or if the provider primes it while it's connected to the patient. This results in the air from the IV tubing entering the patient; that's been in literature quite a few times. In one

case the nurse primed the IV tubing of a two year old baby. He or she gave the child over 30 ccs of air. The baby immediately turned blue and died. After he died, right while the baby was still in the bed, the providers did an x-ray and they could see the air pockets in the brain and in the heart.

If the patient gets a 30 ml block of air in the venous system (picture that in a vein traveling into the heart) it actually fills up the right ventricle with air. This displaces the blood. The air acts as a block. As the blood is flowing through the heart it can't get past the air block. The emergency treatment is to turn the patient on the left side to get that air to rise to the top of the right atrium, which allows the blood to pass through.

3.   The opening in the venous system has to be above heart level; that's a critical factor. Air embolism is not as common in IVs in arms because most IVs are started from the elbow down. They are usually below heart level. But in central lines they are usually in the chest or neck. Jugular lines are very high risk for air embolism on insertion and on maintenance. Nurses who insert jugular IVs have to know that during the procedure when they are taking the wires out and putting the catheters in, there is a direct opening right into the venous system that's above heart level and air can get in pretty quickly. Nurses who maintain the lines need to know that simply changing the tubing or changing the cap can put the patient at risk for air embolism and if the catheter falls out, the patient has an opening above heart level.

4.   The patient must increase his intrathoracic pressure. How do patients do that? This is accomplished by laughing, coughing, sneezing, yelling, crying, hiccupping or simply sighing. It can cause a change in the pressure and that causes air to be sucked into the venous system in a matter of seconds. Patients must be still when the central line is inserted or removed. In one case, after the patient died of an air embolism, the nurse defendant was asked, "How did you remove the line?" She explained how she and the patient were really friendly and in the process of removing the central line she was telling him a very funny joke. During the removal the man was laughing. The nurse did not realize that that was a major contributory factor to the air embolism event. The jury found her negligent. There is a lot of education that needs to be done both from a nursing and medical perspective. Many providers do not realize that this can happen. Air embolism can occur quickly with such serious negative events.

Symptoms of Air Embolism
   If a patient has one of these risk factors that could cause an air embolism what kinds of clinical changes would the healthcare providers see? Surprisingly, there may be few, giving rise to air embolism's nickname as the "silent killer". There is very little documentation in literature about how many air emboli occur every year because people miss it very easily - the symptoms are vague. There may be changes in blood pressure and elevated pulse. Occasionally patients have chest pain and shortness of breath if the air has entered the pulmonary vein. An air embolism in the brain can cause seizures and stroke-like symptoms.

Air within the heart may cause a heart attack. Patients sometimes become confused or disoriented. They may have a "feeling of impending doom"; they feel something is wrong. They don't know exactly what. They may feel fatigued, have a bluish tone to the skin, an irregular heartbeat or breathing, or blurred vision.

When the patient gets enough air into his venous system, death can happen in minutes. It's very quick. According to the literature you may receive 200 ccs of air through a 14 gauge catheter in a second. That's way more than you need to kill somebody. To put that in perspective, a unit of packed red blood cells is about 250 ccs. That's the equivalent of almost a unit of blood.

Detection
A diagnostic study of a brain should show the presence of air. There are CT scans that have positively diagnosed air embolism and formed the basis of many malpractice cases. Air may be present on a CT scan of the brain or in the lung or in the heart. The images will show areas of density on the scan that clearly reveal the size of the air pocket. Prior to the development of a CT scan, the only way pathologists could absolutely diagnose air embolism was on autopsy. The pathologist would open the brain under water to see if air bubbles would come out.

Management of Air Embolism
Saving a patient's life depends on quick recognition and quick treatment of this life-threatening problem. The patient should be turned on her left side so that the air pocket will rise to the top of the right atrium or the right ventricle of the heart. The patient's head should be lowered with her feet elevated. That will also keep the air in the top of the right atrium. If

the patient is fortunate enough to be in a facility that can perform an emergency scan, the radiologist can set up a fluoroscopy machine to identify the location of the air pocket. The physician inserts a needle to suck out the air. In the best scenario, the patient survives without damage. However, in the cases that reach an attorney's desk, the outcome is invariably either death or a vegetative (comatose) state for a lengthy period.

Chapter 16 Liability for Air Embolism

There are two components of liability: the person who allowed the air to get in, and the person responsible for diagnosing and treating the air embolism.

Management of Equipment
IV therapy standards of care address the equipment-related risk factors for air embolism. For example, consider the end caps (that they put on the end of the catheters). The standard of care has been quite clear since a 1991 lawsuit. All connections have to be Luer-locked. (A Luer lock has a thread on it so the cap cannot be removed without twisting it off. In the past it was possible to slip the tubing or the cap into the catheter. This is referred to as "Luer slip".)

The Joint Commission, Infusion Nurses Society Standards of Practice, and the CDC intravascular guidelines all clearly state that all IV connections must be of the Luer-locking type. It should screw on to help minimize the opportunity for the catheter or the tubing or the cap just to slip out. However, Luer-slip tubing is still in use, but it is a huge risk to use those. The manufacturers offer both lines because some anesthesiologists still prefer to use a slip as opposed to a locking connection. The manufacturers offer both types in order to be able to market to the anesthesiologists who want a Luer slip. Even though the force of the standard of care is to use safety needle devices for IV catheters, there are non-safety IV catheters on the market because some anesthesiologists insist upon buying only non-safety devices for inserting IVs.

It is rare for the manufacturing process to create a hole in the catheter. There could be a defect in the catheter material that caused air to get in. Most of the time healthcare providers inadvertently create a hole when they put clamps on the external portion of the catheter or they use a slip clamp. Sometimes when they are changing the dressing, they use scissors and they inadvertently cut the catheter. Med League assisted an attorney by locating an expert witness for a case that involved an air embolism. A nurse used scissors to cut away a dressing and cut a hole in the catheter or clipped the catheter in half to sufficiently damage it. Air entered the system with very poor results for the patient; the suit was settled. A patient may become aggressive and actually cut a catheter with scissors for whatever reason, although a rare event.

Removal of Equipment
There are specific precautions that should be followed when that central catheter is removed from the vein. There is a very specific standard of practice that needs to be followed; it has been in effect since 2000. The Infusion Nurse Society has standards of practice that clearly state the process for how a central venous catheter should be removed. Only trained nurses can remove PICC lines or triple lumen catheters if hospital policy permits. Nurses tend to think that bleeding is the number one risk when they are removing a central venous catheter – which, in fact, it is not, it is the air embolism.

The provider instructs the patient to turn his or her face away and bear down when the tube is removed.

This is the Valsalva maneuver, the process of engaging the patient to stabilize chest pressure. That helps to prevent air from going into the venous system. The patient takes a deep breath, bears down, and holds her breath. While she is in that maneuver, the provider removes the catheter and that stabilizes the pressure and prevents air from going in. Once the nurse applies ointment over the exit site, the patient can breathe normally.

Attorneys questioning defendants involved in an air embolism case may ask, "What do you do when you remove a central line?" The defendant may tell the attorney he puts a Band-Aid over the catheter exit site, whereas the standard says that the healthcare provider should apply an air *occlusive* (prevents air entry) dressing. Some providers think that transparent dressings are air occlusive; they are not. They are air *permeable*. The provider must use something underneath the dressing to make it occlusive. The standard is specific. It is that there must be a gel-based antiseptic that needs to be applied over the catheter exit site - the whole catheter exit site - to prevent air from entering and a transparent dressing put on top of that. But hospital policies may lack specificity and provide inadequate guidance for its staff. Hospital policies may state the staff should use an occlusive dressing on the central line exit site but are not specific about what that is.

Attorneys questioning defendants in an air embolism case may ask, "What type of dressing do you apply?" Nurses may respond they put on gauze and tape. Both are porous. Neither is occlusive. The attorney need not ask defendants how many strips of tape they put on and how long the tape is. Gauze and tape are not occlusive. The standard is specific. An air occlusive dressing is a gel-based ointment and a transparent dressing.

The catheter exit site should be inspected every 24 hours until epithelialization of the skin is evident. In simple terms, that's a scab. When there is scab formation, there is sufficient coverage of the exit site to prevent air from entering. Until the scab is documented as present, the ointment and transparent dressing must be applied. It takes about 72-hours for the scab to form.

Accidental Removal
If the patient accidentally pulls the catheter out, there has to be some emergency equipment at the bedside. There should be ointment at the bedside for some kind of occlusive dressing that the nurse can apply. The attorney may ask a defendant nurse, "What do you do when you walk into a patient's room and the catheter is on the floor? Are you going to walk down the hall and get the ointment?" The nurse has to prevent the air from going in and use a finger, the glove or whatever to prevent that air from going in because air can go into the venous system extremely fast.

Confused patients may pull on their tubes and accidentally remove them. From a liability perspective, when the patient is injured by removing the tube, focus on prevention. What did the staff do to protect the patient from self injury?

- Was there a sitter at the bedside?
- Was there documentation of the sitter being there?
- How often did the nurse come into the room?

- What was the nurse assessing for?
- Was the family notified of the confusion?
- Should the patient's hands have been restrained?

Those kinds of issues have played a very important role in these cases where patients have pulled out intravenous catheters.

Liability Analysis: Diagnosis and Treatment

These are some questions that delve into the liability. There are two issues: how did the air embolism occur? When was it diagnosed?

1. Was there some kind of precipitating event that led the providers to suspect air embolism?
2. Was the air injected or pumped in?
3. Did the air enter during a dressing change?
4. What kind of symptoms did the patient present with?
5. Did the patient's medical record show any definitive documentation there was an air embolism?
6. Was the diagnosis based on symptoms and the event, the time of the event like during a dressing change or during a tubing change?
7. What is the evidence that an air embolism occurred?
8. Should the providers have suspected the air embolism occurred?
9. Did the providers find air in the patient's body?
10. How quickly did the providers recognize the symptoms?
11. How quickly did the providers act to treat the patient?

Defense of Air Embolism Cases

In the absence of a definitive diagnosis, the defense's best hope is to dispute the causation. The neurological expert should address alternative causes for the events associated with the change in the patient's condition.

Complexities of Air Embolism Cases

From a legal perspective, these cases can be difficult to win if there is no hard evidence that shows there was air in the venous system. From a clinical perspective, air emboli are difficult because they happen rapidly and sometimes without the healthcare practitioner even thinking about the risks associated with whatever actions are being taken.

There are few statistics on the amount of air embolism cases because they are frequently not recognized or correctly diagnosed. Many healthcare providers are not aware of the symptoms and they fail to associate the cause (disconnection of tubing) and effect (the patient becomes unconscious and dies). Education is key for nursing and medicine. Definitely, there is a lack of awareness.

Key Points

1. The majority of the focus of IV care is to prevent air embolism.
2. Healthcare providers have to be very knowledgeable about handling IV catheters and tubing. Once there is a disconnection they have to react immediately because air can get in very fast. Once the air gets in, there is very little that they can do.

3.   Rapid diagnosis and treatment is the patient's only hope for any type of reasonable recovery from this devastating type of injury.

The final sections of this book discuss the never event of intravenous catheter-associated blood infections.

Chapter 17 IV Catheter Sepsis

There are a lot more cases of IV catheter-related sepsis than there are of air embolism. In the United States, 15 million central vascular catheter (CVC) days (i.e., the total number of days of exposure to CVCs among all patients in the selected population during the selected time period) occur in intensive care units (ICUs) each year. Studies have variously addressed catheter-related bloodstream infections (CRBSI). These infections independently increase hospital costs and length of stay. While 80,000 CRBSIs occur in ICUs each year, a total of 250,000 cases of BSIs have been estimated to occur annually, if entire hospitals are assessed. By several analyses, the cost of these infections is substantial, both in terms of morbidity and financial resources expended. [8]

Catheter-related sepsis can be extremely serious both clinically and financially. A central line infection that allows bacteria to multiply in the blood stream must be treated with powerful and expensive antibiotics. The development of methicillin resistant staphylococcus aureas (MRSA) and vancomycin resistant enterococcus (VRE) means that many of the commonly used antibiotics are ineffective against these bacteria. Patients can require 6, 8, 9 weeks of antibiotics. Sometimes they do well and that's all they need. But sometimes people can develop really significant negative outcomes. They can have all kinds of side effects from those septicemias. They can be in intensive care units for weeks or months. Sometimes they go into respiratory distress. They could have

---

[8] http://www.cdc.gov/hicpac/BSI/01-BSI-guidelines-2011.html

blood disorders. The infection may travel into organs, where they become virulent. Some patients who are in a compromised state really do not survive those events at all.

Patients may rely on a central line for intravenous nutrition or chemotherapy. The interruption of treatment when that line has to be removed may affect the patient's prognosis. There can be devastating effects if they lose their line and there is a delay in their ability to restart the chemotherapy. Tumor growth becomes an issue in cancer patients. Electrolyte imbalance and nutritional imbalance may result in patients who rely on the line for nutrition. If there is a break in the administration of the medications or solutions, the patient can revert back or have recurrence of symptoms which will ultimately require longer treatment. That's always a big issue in these lawsuits.

The CMS identified 29,536 cases of IV catheter related infections in 2007, at an average cost of $103,027 per hospitalization. Vascular catheter associated infections ranked third in frequency, after pressure sores and preventable injuries such as fractures, dislocations, and burns in 2007, leading to the CMS's decision to stop paying for treatment for a hospital acquired central or peripheral vascular infection as of October 1, 2008. The U. S. Government said, "We are not going to pay for any of that any longer."

Symptoms of IV Sepsis
The most significant symptom is a fever spike above 100.4° with or without drainage from the catheter exit site. Drainage, redness and tenderness at

the site are late signs. Coagulase negative *staphylococci* and Staph aureus are the bacteria that cause the most blood stream infections in all patients. The bacteria normally live on our skin, causing no harm at all. They are a common contaminant of blood stream cultures as they can enter the sampling bottles from the skin. They can cause infections in intravenous lines and of the heart valves (endocarditis, particularly in patients who are already compromised by other medical conditions and treatments).

Enterococci live in the bowel and are increasingly resistant to many antibiotics, including Vancomycin. A study of outbreaks of infections in neonatal ICUs (NICU) showed that the organisms most often involved were klebsiella, and staphylococci, including MRSA. Blood stream infections were the most common type of healthcare associated infection in the NICU.

Culturing the catheters is important for diagnosis of sepsis. The provider who suspects the catheter is infected should be drawing blood cultures through the catheter, so they can identify a specific organism to determine if the catheter is infected. If the catheter is removed they should culture the tip of the catheter to be able to identify if any organisms are on that as well. That helps to determine the catheter was definitely infected or septic as opposed to just basing it on white blood cell counts.

Risk Factors
There is a higher risk of infection with both jugular and femoral central lines. It is harder to maintain a dressing on the neck because patients move their neck, nose, throat and mouth. If they have a

tracheostomy tube, their drainage is in close proximity to the jugular IV site. So it increases the risk of infection.

A femoral line in the groin is hard to keep clean. They are known to have a very, very high infection rate. Patient safety organizations such as the Centers for Disease Control and the Institute for Healthcare Improvement say that femoral lines should be the last choice and used mostly in emergency situations. Residents like to put them in because they are easy to insert. They are a very poor catheter choice from the standpoint of keeping the site clean and what is best for the patient.

Patients at particularly high risk for a blood stream infection include those with diminished immune systems, critically ill patients and neonates. Critically ill patients are at high risk for infection due to altered skin integrity secondary to vascular access. Their lines are frequently manipulated for medication administration. They often have impaired compensatory mechanisms with difficulty combating infection. An infection in a critically ill patient further taxes an already compromised system. Sepsis is the leading cause of death in noncardiac ICUs. Of the 750,000 patients who develop severe sepsis, about one third of them will die. It is estimated that 90% of the deaths due to blood stream infections originate from central venous catheters.

A hospitalized neonate is at high likelihood for needing indwelling catheters and prolonged parenteral nutrition. The infants are particularly susceptible hosts due to the immaturity of their immune system, their low birth weight, and the use of invasive devices and antibiotics. There is an average of 24 patients involved in every outbreak of infection in a NICU.

Significantly more neonates with blood stream infections weigh less than 1,000 grams as compared to neonates who do not develop blood stream infections. Neonates with blood stream infections are more likely to have had a central venous catheter, surgery, been on a ventilator, been on nasal cannula CPAP (continuous positive airway pressure) and a longer mean length of stay. The presence of a central venous catheter is the greatest risk factor. Infants with a catheter have a 9.3 fold increased risk of developing a blood stream infection. The catheters may be manipulated many times a day for administration of fluids, drugs, and blood products. Sometimes catheters may be inserted in urgent situations, during which optimal attention to aseptic technique is challenging.

Prevention

In 2011, the Centers for Disease Control defined the guidelines [9] for prevention of blood stream infections. Below is the summary of their recommendations. The recommendations focus on these main areas:

1. educating and training healthcare personnel who insert and maintain catheters;
2. using maximal sterile barrier precautions during central venous catheter insertion;
3. using a greater than 0.5% chlorhexidine skin preparation with alcohol for antisepsis;
4. avoiding routine replacement of central venous

---

[9] http://www.cdc.gov/hicpac/BSI/01-BSI-guidelines-2011.html

5.   catheters as a strategy to prevent infection; and
6.   using antiseptic/antibiotic impregnated short-term central venous catheters and chlorhexidine impregnated sponge dressings if the rate of infection is not decreasing despite adherence to other strategies (i.e., education and training, maximal sterile barrier precautions, and greater than 0.5% chlorhexidine preparations with alcohol for skin antisepsis).

Each recommendation is categorized on the basis of existing scientific data, theoretical rationale, applicability, and economic impact. The system for categorizing recommendations in this guideline is as follows:

Category IA. Strongly recommended for implementation and strongly supported by well-designed experimental, clinical, or epidemiologic studies.

Category IB. Strongly recommended for implementation and supported by some experimental, clinical, or epidemiologic studies and a strong theoretical rationale; or an accepted practice (e.g., aseptic technique) supported by limited evidence.

Category IC. Required by state or federal regulations, rules, or standards.

Category II. Suggested for implementation and supported by suggestive clinical or epidemiologic studies or a theoretical rationale. This is an unresolved issue for which evidence is insufficient or no consensus regarding efficacy exists.

Education, Training and Staffing

1.   Educate healthcare personnel regarding the indications for intravascular catheter use, proper procedures for the insertion and maintenance of intravascular catheters, and appropriate infection control measures to prevent intravascular catheter-related infections. Category IA

2.   Periodically assess knowledge of and adherence to guidelines for all personnel involved in the insertion and maintenance of intravascular catheters. Category IA

3.   Designate only trained personnel who demonstrate competence for the insertion and maintenance of peripheral and central intravascular catheters. Category IA

4.   Ensure appropriate nursing staff levels in ICUs. Observational studies suggest that a higher proportion of "pool nurses" or an elevated patient–to-nurse ratio is associated with CRBSI in ICUs where nurses are managing patients with CVCs. Category IB

Selection of Catheters and Sites: Peripheral Catheters and Midline Catheters

1.   In adults, use an upper-extremity site for catheter insertion. Replace a catheter inserted in a lower extremity site to an upper extremity site as soon as possible. Category II

2.   In pediatric patients, the upper or lower extremities or the scalp (in neonates or young infants) can be used as the catheter insertion site. Category II

3.   Select catheters on the basis of the intended purpose and duration of use, known infectious and non-infectious complications (e.g., phlebitis

and infiltration), and experience of individual catheter operators. Category IB
4. Avoid the use of steel needles for the administration of fluids and medication that might cause tissue necrosis if extravasation occurs. Category IA
5. Use a midline catheter or peripherally inserted central catheter (PICC), instead of a short peripheral catheter, when the duration of IV therapy will likely exceed six days. Category II
6. Evaluate the catheter insertion site daily by palpation through the dressing to discern tenderness and by inspection if a transparent dressing is in use. Gauze and opaque dressings should not be removed if the patient has no clinical signs of infection. If the patient has local tenderness or other signs of possible CRBSI, an opaque dressing should be removed and the site inspected visually. Category II
7. Remove peripheral venous catheters if the patient develops signs of phlebitis (warmth, tenderness, erythema or palpable venous cord), infection, or a malfunctioning catheter. Category IB

Central Venous Catheters
1. Weigh the risks and benefits of placing a central venous device at a recommended site to reduce infectious complications against the risk for mechanical complications (e.g., pneumothorax, subclavian artery puncture, subclavian vein laceration, subclavian vein stenosis, hemothorax, thrombosis, air embolism, and catheter misplacement). Category IA
2. Avoid using the femoral vein for central venous access in adult patients. Category 1A

3. Use a subclavian site, rather than a jugular or a femoral site, in adult patients to minimize infection risk for nontunneled CVC placement. Category IB
4. No recommendation can be made for a preferred site of insertion to minimize infection risk for a tunneled CVC. Unresolved issue
5. Avoid the subclavian site in hemodialysis patients and patients with advanced kidney disease, to avoid subclavian vein stenosis. Category IA
6. Use a fistula or graft in patients with chronic renal failure instead of a CVC for permanent access for dialysis. Category 1A
7. Use ultrasound guidance to place central venous catheters (if this technology is available) to reduce the number of cannulation attempts and mechanical complications. Ultrasound guidance should only be used by those fully trained in its technique. Category 1B
8. Use a CVC with the minimum number of ports or lumens essential for the management of the patient. Category IB
9. No recommendation can be made regarding the use of a designated lumen for parenteral nutrition. Unresolved issue
10. Promptly remove any intravascular catheter that is no longer essential. Category IA
11. When adherence to aseptic technique cannot be ensured (i.e catheters inserted during a medical emergency), replace the catheter as soon as possible, i.e, within 48 hours. Category IB

Hand Hygiene and Aseptic Technique
1. Perform hand hygiene procedures, either by washing hands with conventional soap and water

or with alcohol-based hand rubs (ABHR). Hand hygiene should be performed before and after palpating catheter insertion sites as well as before and after inserting, replacing, accessing, repairing, or dressing an intravascular catheter. Palpation of the insertion site should not be performed after the application of antiseptic, unless aseptic technique is maintained. Category IB

2. Maintain aseptic technique for the insertion and care of intravascular catheters. Category IB
3. Wear clean gloves, rather than sterile gloves, for the insertion of peripheral intravascular catheters, if the access site is not touched after the application of skin antiseptics. Category IC
4. Sterile gloves should be worn for the insertion of arterial, central, and midline catheters. Category IA
5. Use new sterile gloves before handling the new catheter when guidewire exchanges are performed. Category II
6. Wear either clean or sterile gloves when changing the dressing on intravascular catheters. Category IC

Maximal Sterile Barrier Precautions
1. Use maximal sterile barrier precautions, including the use of a cap, mask, sterile gown, sterile gloves, and a sterile full body drape, for the insertion of CVCs, PICCs, or guidewire exchange. Category IB
2. Use a sterile sleeve to protect pulmonary artery catheters during insertion. Category IB

Skin Preparation

1. Prepare clean skin with an antiseptic (70% alcohol, tincture of iodine, or alcoholic chlorhexidine gluconate solution) before peripheral venous catheter insertion. Category IB

2. Prepare clean skin with a >0.5% chlorhexidine preparation with alcohol before central venous catheter and peripheral arterial catheter insertion and during dressing changes. If there is a contraindication to chlorhexidine, tincture of iodine, an iodophor, or 70% alcohol can be used as alternatives. Category IA

3. No comparison has been made between using chlorhexidine preparations with alcohol and providone-iodine in alcohol to prepare clean skin. Unresolved issue.

4. No recommendation can be made for the safety or efficacy of chlorhexidine in infants aged less than 2 months. Unresolved issue

5. Antiseptics should be allowed to dry according to the manufacturer's recommendation prior to placing the catheter. Category IB

Catheter Site Dressing Regimens

1. Use either sterile gauze or sterile, transparent, semipermeable dressing to cover the catheter site. Category IA

2. If the patient is diaphoretic or if the site is bleeding or oozing, use a gauze dressing until this is resolved. Category II

3. Replace catheter site dressing if the dressing becomes damp, loosened, or visibly soiled. Category IB

4. Do not use topical antibiotic ointment or creams on insertion sites, except for dialysis catheters,

because of their potential to promote fungal infections and antimicrobial resistance. Category IB

5. Do not submerge the catheter or catheter site in water. Showering should be permitted if precautions can be taken to reduce the likelihood of introducing organisms into the catheter (e.g., if the catheter and connecting device are protected with an impermeable cover during the shower). Category IB

6. Replace dressings used on short-term CVC sites every 2 days for gauze dressings. Category II

7. Replace dressings used on short-term CVC sites at least every 7 days for transparent dressings, except in those pediatric patients in which the risk for dislodging the catheter may outweigh the benefit of changing the dressing. Category IB

8. Replace transparent dressings used on tunneled or implanted CVC sites no more than once per week (unless the dressing is soiled or loose), until the insertion site has healed. Category II

9. No recommendation can be made regarding the necessity for any dressing on well-healed exit sites of long-term cuffed and tunneled CVCs. Unresolved issue

10. Ensure that catheter site care is compatible with the catheter material. Category IB

11. Use a sterile sleeve for all pulmonary artery catheters. Category IB

12. Use a chlorhexidine-impregnated sponge dressing for temporary short-term catheters in patients older than 2 months of age if the CLABSI rate is not decreasing despite adherence to basic prevention measures, including education and training, appropriate use of

chlorhexidine for skin antisepsis, and MSB. Category 1B

13. No recommendation is made for other types of chlorhexidine dressings. Unresolved issue

14. Monitor the catheter sites visually when changing the dressing or by palpation through an intact dressing on a regular basis, depending on the clinical situation of the individual patient. If patients have tenderness at the insertion site, fever without obvious source, or other manifestations suggesting local or bloodstream infection, the dressing should be removed to allow thorough examination of the site. Category IB

15. Encourage patients to report any changes in their catheter site or any new discomfort to their provider. Category II [10]

Changing Procedures

It's a slow process, in terms of disseminating information about intravenous catheter standards of care and making sure that facilities are purchasing the correct equipment and empowering staff to insist upon these changes. There are so many components that go into this. Staff members have to be more attentive to washing their hands than they have been in the past because of the link between poor hand hygiene and catheter-related infections. Staff members have to speak up when they see a colleague who has omitted washing her hands. This takes courage and a willingness to engage in confrontation.

---

[10]http://www.cdc.gov/hicpac/BSI/02-bsi-summary-of-recommendations-2011.html

I heard a discussion at a patient safety conference about the concept of empowering staff to stop the procedure if they saw a break in technique or improper use of equipment. The term was "stop the line." The analogy is like stopping the factory line if you see some defect slipping through. Stop the line in this context refers to stopping the procedure. Some of the central line insertion trays come with stop signs. The assistant, usually a nurse, is able to hold up the sign. He or she should put that sign up and say, "Stop, step away from the patient. We need to get a new set up."

Some hospital staff spend a great deal of effort to reeducate the staff on hand washing and teaching what happens when they don't wash their hands properly. They post signs in the facility to remind people to wash their hands frequently. This often results in significant improvement in hand washing techniques. They also find that if they do not repeat that education on an ongoing basis that the numbers slide right back to what they were before the training. Education and reeducation of the staff is important when it comes to proper hand washing techniques.

Healthcare providers should wash their hands:

- When they are obviously soiled
- Before and after invasive procedures
- Between patients
- After removing gloves
- Before and after eating
- After using the bathroom
- If contamination is suspected

Can education make a difference? In a study sponsored by the AHRQ (Agency for Healthcare

Research and Quality), Peter Pronovost and associates examined the impact of implementing CDC guidelines on the catheter related blood stream infection rate in ICUs in Michigan. Infection rates were measured at 3 month intervals up to 18 months after implementation. The 103 hospitals reporting data found at 16-18 months after implementation, the mean catheter related blood stream infection rate decreased by 66% when compared with the rate before the study. Conference calls, quarterly meetings and daily goal sheets were used to track progress in these hospitals.

Just wearing gloves is not enough. Some healthcare staff wear the same gloves all day, thinking that by wearing the gloves, they don't need to wash their hands as frequently. But they have to change their gloves in between each patient and wash their hands even if they are wearing gloves in between each patient. From a sepsis point of view, all these things can be the cause of the infection. I came across the startling statistic that MRSA can live on the surfaces of curtains and counters and table tops for 11 days. Think about a nurse changing the dressing that's contaminated with MRSA and then instead of removing the gloves, reaching out and pushing the curtain aside. He has just transferred the organism onto the curtains waiting for somebody else to come along and pick it up.

For preventing IV catheter-related sepsis, sterile technique on insertion of the catheter is of the utmost concern. Sterile trays and maximum barrier precautions are now required, which means the patient needs to be draped with sterile drapes from head to toe before the catheter can be inserted. Also, the use of Chlorhexidine is very important for cleaning the site. The inserter has to be in a gown, a mask, goggles and hair cover. That is the requirement now from the IHI, The Joint Commission and the CDC. The inserter needle can only be used once. If the physician or the nurse misses, they need to get a new needle. They cannot reuse the same needle.

The medical community recommends that doctors should not be inserting these central lines by use of land marking. They should be using bedside ultrasound so that they can clearly identify the vein that they are sticking so that they can get the vein on the first attempt as opposed to doing all that probing. So, all those factors will help to decrease the opportunity for sepsis, or catheter-related sepsis.

Chapter 18 Liability for IV Catheter Infections

The phone rings in the plaintiff attorney's office and the caller says, "My husband died of a blood stream infection in the hospital". From the liability perspective, if a plaintiff attorney has a case or is being approached by a family with a case involving an IV catheter line, these are some suggestions for medical record review to determine if there is liability.

1. Look at the medical record to see if the healthcare professionals have written the diagnosis of catheter-related sepsis.
2. Look to see if there were any blood cultures or catheter tip cultures done.
3. Look at the IV insertion sheet if there is any. When was the IV put in and when did the providers first suspect that the patient may have had a septic catheter? It takes a lot of detective work to find out in the chart if there really is a catheter-related sepsis.

Plaintiff attorneys are increasingly aware of the whole concept of never events and are looking at these issues in terms of whether or not they can establish that there is liability associated with the development of that infection. However, it's very difficult to determine a liability or negligence with a catheter related infection. The courts are very specific; they want to know how it happened and precisely when it happened and what is the evidence of those two factors. It's really very hard to pinpoint exactly when it happened and that's the issue for infections or catheter related infections. Here are some additional considerations, which will be difficult to establish retroactively.

- Was the patient's infection insertion-related?
- Did the doctor fail to use proper sterile technique when she was putting the line in?
- Was it a nursing error because they didn't change the dressing properly or they didn't change the tubing properly?
- Was the patient manipulating the line? (The nurses may chart this.)
- What was the patient's condition? The patient can be really debilitated or immunocompromised, such as a cancer patient who has a very low white count and is very susceptible to infection.

Once the IV catheter infection was identified, was the appropriate treatment ordered? It's easier to establish liability if the appropriate organism was identified but the incorrect antibiotic was ordered or an incorrect frequency or dosing of the antibiotic was ordered.

- If there was a culture, which antibiotic was the organism sensitive to?
- How soon was the antibiotic ordered? Did they wait 48 hours? Did they wait 24 hours? Did they start it right away? The delay in treatment is always a big issue.
- Was the patient monitored during the treatment with IV antibiotics, to make sure that they were effective?
- Was the dose high enough? Was it low enough?
- Was the frequency appropriate?

- Was it given on time?

Did the facility provide an environment that supported infection avoidance? Did they

- assess barriers to washing hands?
- reinforce the behavior through observations?
- use posters in bathrooms?
- include hand hygiene in a checklist for central line insertion?
- keep equipment such as soap/alcohol based dispensers in convenient locations?
- measure rates of compliance?
- post signs in the patient room as reminders to wash hands?
- provide educational and awareness campaigns for both healthcare workers and patients to improve compliance with hand hygiene?
- hold staff accountable for hand hygiene?
- teach patients to speak up if their providers did not wash their hands?
- provide chlorhexidrine?
- perform a daily review of central line necessity to prevent unnecessary delays in removing lines that are no longer necessary?
- ensure that all staff who insert lines, including physicians, document the time and date of insertion?
- ask on daily rounds why the central line is still in place and whether it is still needed?
- comply with other aspects of the CDC recommendations cited above?

Defenses

It is very hard to pinpoint that one event that was the cause or the source of the catheter-related infection. It is very easy to get these infections but hard to pinpoint how it happened.

Defense experts may argue there are things that the healthcare clinician can really not control. The patient will have a catheter-related sepsis if the patient is immunocompromised - if the patient has a history of cancer or has a very low white count, like transplant patients, oncology patients who are immunocompromised - those patients are very high risk for sepsis. Even with the best care, it may not be possible to prevent catheter-related sepsis. The patients' white blood cell counts are so low they are not able to fight off even the smallest bacterial invasion. The condition of the patient is the big issue from the defense perspective.

This is a big concern because central catheters are typically used in people who are in an immunocompromised state. There are multiple manipulations of the tubing to give medications and fluids. So there is a lot of opportunity for quite unintentionally introducing organisms into the system.

However, CMS will deny reimbursement for hospital acquired IV sepsis even for those immunocompromised patients. There was a lot of controversy related to putting IV catheter-related sepsis on the list of non-reimbursable conditions. Yet, if it had a positive effect in terms of improving people's perspective or changing performance on these issues it can only be of greater value to healthcare consumers. The number of hospital acquired catheter- related sepsis infections is way too high and the only way you are going to get a hospital's attention is to say to them, "We are not going to pay for the treatment."

Key Points

1. Blood infections caused by intravenous equipment or breaks in sterile technique may cause life-threatening infections.
2. Handwashing is an essential but often neglected part of delivering medical and nursing care.
3. Many patients are at high risk for intravenous infections, including neonates, the elderly and critically ill.
4. It is often easier to allege a delay in diagnosis of infection, a delay in starting antibiotic therapy, or ordering the incorrect therapy than to determine who infected the patient.

Conclusion

The majority of this text has focused on never events – ones that may lead to high treatment cost, prolonged suffering, and denied reimbursement for hospital care. Falls, pressure sores, air embolism and intravenous extravasation may ultimately result in the patient's death. Healthcare providers are increasingly aware of the clinical and financial risks associated with the development of these never events. Attorneys are increasingly seeing plaintiffs alleging deviations from the standard of care related to these events.

This text was designed to provide the attorney and legal nurse consultant with concrete guidance on the causes, damages, prevention and liability aspects associated with these events.

Obtain legal nurse consulting resources at www.legalnursebusiness.com.

Consider Writing a Review

Thank you for buying this book. When you enjoy a book, it is a natural desire to tell others about it. Amazon.com provides a way to share your thoughts and I invite you to write a book review. It is easy. Here are tips:

1. After going to the link below on Amazon.com, the first thing you are asked to do is to assign a number of stars to the book you think matches your opinion of the book.
2. Create a title for the review. This can be a simple phrase, like "Awesome guide." If you are not sure what to say, look at the titles of other book reviews.
3. It is easiest to write the book in a word processor and then paste it into Amazon.com Your word processor will pick up typos before your review goes public.
4. Write the review as if you were talking to another person – you are – a person who comes to Amazon.com and is considering buying this book.
5. Include a description of what you found most helpful. Was it an idea, chapter, tip? Share that with the readers.
6. Next you may want to write who you think would most benefit from this book. Is it for beginners? Or is it more appropriate for someone with experience with this topic?
7. What if you have something negative to say about the book? You may always reach me at patriciaiyer@gmail.com to suggest changes in the book.
8. If you include negative feedback in the review, keep a positive perspective rather than attack the author.

Here are some sample phrases:

- - While overall the book was good, I would change it by. . .
- - I don't think this book is right for. . .
- - I would improve this book by. . .

Before you hit save, read everything over one more time.

Authors and readers appreciate book reviews and they get easier to write with time. Go to this link on Amazon.com to write your review. If for any reason it does not work, search for the book title + Iyer and it will show.

Link: http://bit.ly/FallsPUIV

Thank you,
Pat Iyer